THE MAN
with NO LEGS

THE MAN
with NO LEGS
"My Journey with God"

Russ Sharrock
and Alice Taylor Sharrock

XULON PRESS

Xulon Press
2301 Lucien Way #415
Maitland, FL 32751
407.339.4217
www.xulonpress.com

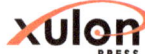

© 2019 by Russ Sharrock

All rights reserved solely by the author. The author guarantees all contents are original and do not infringe upon the legal rights of any other person or work. No part of this book may be reproduced in any form without the permission of the author. The views expressed in this book are not necessarily those of the publisher.

Unless otherwise indicated, Scripture quotations taken from the Holy Bible, New International Version (NIV). Copyright © 1973, 1978, 1984, 2011 by Biblica, Inc.™. Used by permission. All rights reserved.

Printed in the United States of America.

ISBN-13: 978-1-6295-2969-1

Table of Contents

†

Foreword vii
Acknowledgments xi
Introduction xiii

1. The Journey Begins 1
2. A New Direction 9
3. Following Our Dream 19
4. Putting Out the Fleece 27
5. Time to Pack Your Bags—Again 35
6. The Next Great Adventure 45
7. Living the Wilderness Life 65
8. The Call of South Asia 79
9. Retirement—Or Is It? 89
10. The Cross Roads of Life 99
11. Return to India 107
12. The Times, They Are Changing 131
13. The Caribbean Call 135

An Invitation to Our Readers 159

Foreword

---†---

When Russ and Alice Sharrock moved to Stillwater, OK, more than 10 years ago they began going to the same church Bob and I were attending as newcomers as well. Being in the same Sunday school class, it soon became clear to us that they were wholeheartedly committed to Jesus Christ and the Great Commission with a deep desire to introduce the Gospel to people everywhere.

Walking down the driveway between a fence and the big black truck (fitted for an amputee to drive) and a good sized camping trailer, I stepped onto the ramp to the small deck and rang the doorbell. "Come on in," came the voice of the man in the wheelchair. I entered and saw a small living room on the left with comfortable rattan cushioned furniture and Russ's desk and computer – his work space. On the right was the kitchen and small dining table.

It was time to enjoy warm fellowship, loud laughter, and story after story of the many places God had taken them, and of the people, characters one and all. From the extreme cold of Alaska, to the crowds and smells of India, to the third world life and heat of Haiti, Russ and Alice made their adventures all come to life.

Their ministry left a trail of changed lives from Idaho to Virginia to Oklahoma. What a delight to be in their home, enjoying their warm hospitality, reliving many of their adventures.

Russ began a non-profit mission and asked me to serve on the board. Our meetings revealed a person who was excited, energetic, and full of vision and ideas, as well as being a man of integrity. Despite the pain of severe medical problems, his vision did not dim although the door to India closed. They had been to India many times often taking teams with them.

When Russ was enduring three amputation surgeries, Alice not only vicariously experienced the terrible pain, but she carried on the business to give them an income and a place to live. Day after day she did the work of two, answering the phone, renting vehicles, cleaning out storage units, etc. God gave her unusual strength to keep them from having nothing. Then God wonderfully provided them with a small Habitat for Humanity home, ideal for their needs.

Russ began to be the facilitator using the M-28 method of Bible study in our church's Friday evening international Bible study. The method was a challenge to him because he had to switch from more direct telling and teaching to asking questions and watching and waiting as the biblical truth came alive to them. This was not what he had been taught in Bible College or seminary. He did learn it, seeing how the Holy Spirit opens the eyes of the blind, putting truth into their hearts. These lessons were a time for the internationals to learn how to do the same thing in their home countries. He and Alice were always opening their home to anyone who would come.

They then began to minister in Haiti under difficult circumstances. Alice Taylor, the artist, used her lifetime of painting, selling, and shows to teach them art. Helping the young Haitians paint their vision, their lives became such a blessing to her. She envisioned these talented young people finding a way to make a living in a very poor environment.

I saw how she was heartbroken when they could no longer live in Haiti. Due to health reasons they could not live under such trying conditions.

As their autobiography reveals they are always pushing ahead with vision and joy, currently starting a new non-profit mission. They are both extraordinarily gifted and are constantly seeking ways to serve Jesus Christ, no matter the cost. They are also adventurous and fun-loving which makes their writing an interesting read.

— Rosalie A. Larzelere–2019

Acknowledgments

———†———

Dozens of people have had an impact on the writing of this book—from those who have urged me to write it, to all those who have influenced my life and ministry through the good times and the bad. I want to thank all of them, especially: William and Becky Gunter, our first pastor and his wife, who initially set my feet on the path of ministry and leadership. Bob and Sandra Jackson, who eased me into preaching without my realizing it. Carroll Fowler, a fellow renegade, who taught me that planting churches and spreading the Gospel works just fine if you do things "outside the box."

Of those who have been especially instrumental in bringing this book to pass during the long writing, editing, and reviewing of this manuscript, I want to thank Rosalie Larzelere for her friendship, encouragement, and her discerning editing skills as she took my writing and smoothed out the rough edges. I would like to thank my High School friend, Judith Palfrey of Palfrey Associates for the wonderful job she did in preparing my photos for the book.

My greatest debt is to my wife and best friend Alice, for her typing and additional comments in the book, editing help, suggestions, and sorting images that has made the crucial difference in bringing a story to life. She has loved me, nursed me, and traveled with me to wherever God has led. A long time ago she learned to always have a suitcase packed and ready to go. Her emotional and spiritual support made the writing of this book possible. I am certain that without her standing beside me and encouraging me during these eventful years, this book and the message it proclaims, would not have been possible. Most of all, thanks to the Lord God Almighty, Who found this black sheep and made me His own, through His Son and my Savior, Jesus Christ.

Introduction

———†———

Just as I did, many of you probably grew up with a favorite Christian book, quite possibly due to the way it challenged you, or how it made you look at the world. For works of fiction, it might be due to an intriguing character or an engaging story.

C.S. Lewis once wrote:

> "Literary experience heals the wound, without undermining the privilege of Individuality. There are mass emotions which heal the wound; but they destroy the privilege. In them our separate selves are pooled and we sink back into Sub-individuality. But in reading great literature I become a thousand men and yet remain myself. Like the night sky in the Greek poem, I see with a myriad eyes, but it is still I who see. Here, as in worship, in love, in moral action, and in knowing, I transcend myself, and am never more myself than when I do." [1]

---

[1] C.S. Lewis, *An Experiment in Criticism,* Cambridge University Press, 1961

Here, Lewis looks at the enormous power writing has to expand our inner world, and how inspirational books also manage to soothe our most overpowering emotions. Those of us who read know there are a number of wonderful characters to whom we can give credit for this pastime. My mom began teaching me to read when I was only three years old. First, were Bible stories of some of the great men and women of faith who trusted God, and He was able to use them throughout the continuing story that ultimately led to the arrival of the Messiah, God's Son and our Savior, Jesus the Christ.

The first Christian book I read for theology and building my faith was the Bible. Considering how pervasive biblical illiteracy is in America today, we should probably focus more on Scripture and fewer current publications. The Bible is a beautiful book inspired by God to give hope to millions and is the ultimate authority for our lives. With the help of Christian books, we can distill certain messages and stories of the Bible to better understand the problems that face us today.

With that being said, my goal in writing "The Man with No Legs" is to help you deepen your faith in the One who is always faithful, "For the word of the LORD is right and true; he is faithful in all he does. The LORD loves righteousness and justice; the earth is full of his unfailing love." (Psalm 33:4-5) My desire is to be an encouragement to you through the times of crisis that invariably occur throughout our lives. I want everyone to understand that God can use the most unlikely people to accomplish His purpose. And God can use the most impossible situations for His glory.

Chapter One

The Journey Begins

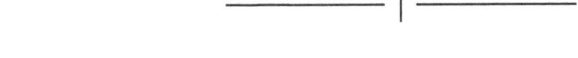

Vincent van Gogh once wrote:

> "It is an old belief and it is a good belief, that our life is a pilgrim's progress – that we are strangers on the earth, but that though this be so, yet we are not alone for our Father is with us. We are pilgrims, our life is a long walk or journey from earth to Heaven." [2]

The fog of anesthesia was slowly lifting and reality began to hit me hard. No longer would I roll out of bed in the morning to greet the day. No longer would I walk in the cool of the evening and hear the quail calling as they went to roost. No longer would I be able to climb mountains or hike through the fields of my beloved outdoors. The freedom and mobility provided by my legs and feet were gone forever. I was now a cripple. The Man with No Legs.

---

[2] Vincent van Gogh's First Sunday Sermon: 29 October 1876

Yet, as I looked back, God had been preparing me for this day. It is an odd feeling sometimes to look back and see footprints running parallel to yours. You think you have everything under control; that you're young, strong and the entire world is before you. Then one day, you come to the realization that you were never really on your own; that there was always someone beside you, ready to catch you when, inevitably, you fell.

I have lived what many might consider an extraordinary life, having walked alongside men who were leaders, slept in the homes of the poor, and crossed continents to bring the good news of the gospel to the world. I'm not sure how best to describe the early years of my life. I was born in 1949 into a military family. I grew up in a Christian family in the fifties and sixties, with a father who worked very hard to provide for us both physically and spiritually.

Our mother gave us the love and nurturing that most kids today only seem to dream about. I am so grateful to them for the life they gave me. Throughout my early years of development my family attended Lexington Park Baptist Church in St. Mary's County, MD, and at the tender age of seven years old I received Jesus as my Savior. Shortly thereafter, I had the privilege of being baptized along with my mother who had recently converted from Catholicism and made a profession of faith in Jesus Christ. To this day, I do not believe I truly understood the full implications of that decision. My mother and I had a closer relationship than I had with my father leading to my eventual belief that I was probably only following my mother's example as she made her way down the aisle of decision.

The Journey Begins

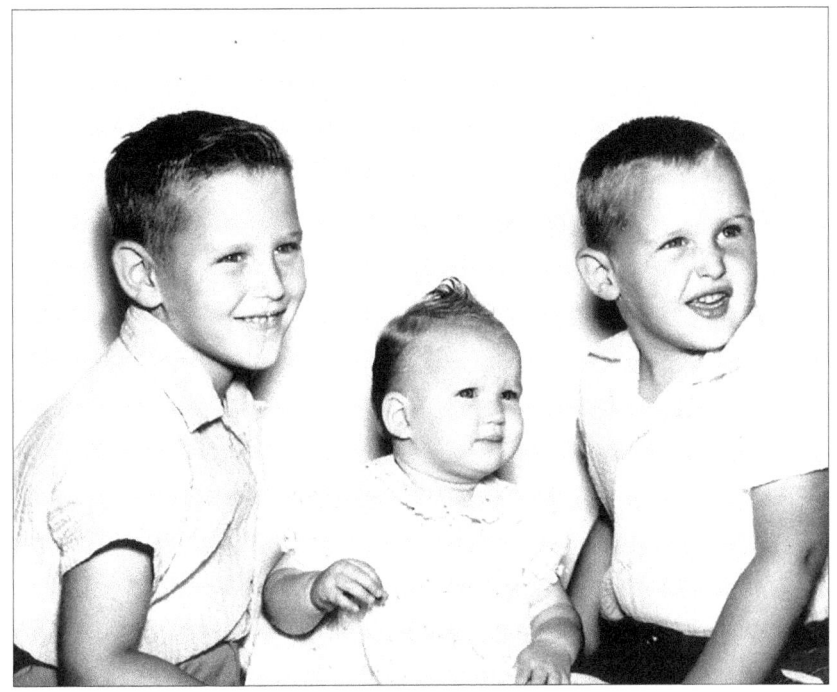

From Left: Russ, Pam, Allan

Even at a fairly young age I thought of myself as a bit of a loner. I had very few friends, none of which could have been considered best friends. And as I entered my teen years I found that sense of loneliness growing deeper and the outdoors became my best friend.

The author Os Guinness in His book *Long Journey Home* observed, "It's often said that there are three requirements for a fulfilling life. The first two—a clear sense of personal identity and a strong sense of personal mission—are rooted in the third: a deep sense of life's meaning." [3] There are many different reasons people give for their search for fulfillment in today's world. Sometimes it is the sense that their life lacks any close

---

[3] Os Guinness, "Long Journey Home," by WaterBrook Press, Page 2, 2001

relationships. They may feel they're trapped in a boring, dead end job, or maybe it is trying to live with some assumed burden of life such as feelings of guilt. I cannot say I ever considered myself to be any kind of philosopher but I clearly had no sense of identity, nor any kind of personal mission in life.

I had a rather uneventful childhood until I reached my teen years. As a teenager, I was young, impulsive, and more than a little immature. Not a good combination. I felt an emptiness and a sense of meaninglessness. I became entangled in the cultural revolution of the sixties and seventies and I rebelled against God, family, and against society, as I began searching for that elusive "something" I felt was missing in my life. And so began my journey.

Since the beginning there have been stories told around campfires, the great halls of castles, and up through today's Hollywood movies with the central idea of life as a journey. In Dante's story, *Divine Comedy*, he writes, "Midway on our life's journey I found myself in a dark wood." So many authors throughout history from the Old Testament book of *Exodus*, John Bunyan's *Pilgrim's Progress*, and Hermann Hesse's *Siddhartha* among others, explored life as a journey or pilgrimage; a journey which all of us are on at some point whether just beginning or approaching its conclusion.

I had the whole world before me and I wanted to see what it had to offer. So I set out to find my own way. From that point on it was a downhill slide. This was the 60's, and the country was well into the counter culture era. A time of hippies, free love, and drugs. And I became deeply enmeshed in that Cultural Revolution very quickly.

My parents were so excited when I decided to follow my father's footsteps into the Navy, and had great hope this would change my perspective on life. It helped somewhat, but not as much as I needed. After the military, I spent many years traveling through life without any idea what I was doing and where I was going. The next nine years were a journey spanning three countries in search of peace, happiness, and contentment, but all I found were drugs, alcohol, and broken dreams. I wandered from one town, one drink, and one relationship to the next. Always wondering what was over the next hill, always seeking that next adventure. But each step I took into what appeared like an exciting new adventure quickly became misery and emptiness. I had such a rebellious attitude I could not find and hold a job for very long. Most of those years were spent on the street trying to "panhandle" enough money for a meal, although most of it went to purchase alcohol and cigarettes. Surprisingly, the easiest to find were drugs. In those days they were much cheaper, and there were always "so-called" friends around who would share a joint or a needle. My "great adventure" saw the years going by without the purpose I was seeking, or anything else for that matter.

Throughout this period of my life, my parents never gave up hope. They believed in the power of prayer and they prayed for me constantly. When I was in town they would always welcome me home. I'll always remember the many times I would go into my bedroom and on my pillow would be a scripture verse or the Bible would be laid open to the story of the Prodigal son. God never gave up hope on me either, but I was not ready to turn my life over to Him.

I still believed I could find my own way in life, and I refused to admit that the life I was finding continued to lead only to nothingness. During those days I hitchhiked extensively across the U.S., up into Canada, and down into Mexico; a job here, a party there. Yet, I was still bored, lonely, and empty, and I tried to fill that emptiness with just about anything that came along.

At one point I even joined a satanic cult for a short period of time. But some of the things I experienced there literally scared me straight. To this day I take the biblical teaching about demons very seriously.

One summer evening in 1973, a friend of mine and I were hanging out on the campus of St Mary's College in Maryland when I received word that my younger brother had been in an automobile accident while serving at the Pensacola Naval Base in Pensacola, Florida. My parents were sitting around the kitchen table with a few close friends from church and waiting for news of my brother's condition. My sister came to pick me up from St Mary's college and we went to be with my parents. Shortly after arriving home, my dad got the phone call that no parent ever wants to receive, Allan had passed away. They were devastated! And my mother almost had a breakdown.

It took a couple of years before she or my father came to grips with the loss of their middle child. A young man who had the world at his feet; a good job as an aircraft mechanic, a beautiful fiancé, and all of life in front of him. On the other hand, my parents had me, the black sheep of the family. A wandering party boy without much hope and no prospects for a job or even a stable relationship. In fact, on the night my brother died our neighbors were conveying their condolences to my parents and expressing how sad it was to lose their son when they said, "He was such a fine young man, if anyone had to die it should have been Russ." Sad to say, that assessment of my life was pretty spot on. And when I overheard that painful statement, instead of turning my life around, I left to hit the road once again.

There is no pride in saying this, but I have probably seen and/or participated in just about every evil and wicked way, short of murder, which exists in the world; and I came very close to that at one time. I have even been through "the valley of the shadow of Death" and wondered for many years how or even why I had survived. This is a part of my story I had never told anyone except my wife, and many years later I finally told my parents.

It was near the end of 1976. I was a moderately heavy drug user and I had recently scored a large quantity of Crystal Meth-Amphetamine and had been high on it for about four days. On the fifth day, I got together with a few of my buddies for a party and decided to take some LSD in a form called Window Pane. It was like a small, clear, flat tablet that was considered pretty pure. We then bought some Tequila to wash it down. Well, actually, several bottles of Tequila. About thirty minutes later my whole body suddenly became numb, and I lost all mobility. It was as if my legs had suddenly disappeared and I collapsed to the floor. The guys carried me to the bedroom and laid me on the bed. I had lost all feeling in my body and could not see anything else in the room except the ceiling tiles above my head. I could still hear them talking. They were trying to decide whether or not to call for an ambulance. They were afraid the police might also show up and they didn't want that. Then one of them said, "I can't feel a pulse; I don't think he's breathing." About that time, I began to feel lighter and the ceiling tiles start coming closer as if I was floating up toward them.

I could no longer hear anyone talking and I felt all alone. I had no sense of time and everything seemed suspended. Then all of a sudden, and I don't know of any way to explain this, but I felt like I was back lying on the bed. I felt fine, so I got up and went into the living room to see everyone. The look on their faces was priceless, as if they had seen a ghost. They said they thought I was dead and were trying to decide how to handle this situation, either dump my body in the woods or maybe just call my parents to come pick it up. Either way, like "true addict friends," they weren't going to stick around. For many days after that incident, I thought about what had happened and even considered the possibility that God had a hand in it. My parents never knew how close they had come to losing another son until many years later. That episode definitely scared me. I had looked death in the face—and maybe it was time to change my ways. I wish I could say I changed right then and there, but it was a long, slow road back. And it was a while before I finally took it.

As the years rolled by, and all the "great adventures" continued to lead nowhere, my parent's love and the scriptures stayed with me. Even though it took another year, I finally broke free of the drugs and cigarettes, but alcohol was another story. I still had a burden of guilt in my life—I had let my parents down, I had let God down, and I had let myself down. Here I was in my late twenties, no job, no education, and—I believed—no hope. I began going to church on and off, but my feeble attempts at jobs and education met with failure. Because of this I often slid back into hiding myself in alcohol. I was fighting to get back to God in my own weak strength and too stubborn to simply turn it completely over to Him. But life went on.

Chapter 2

A New Direction

———†———

It was now 1987. I was thirty-eight years old and desperately needed a job. Thanks to the influence of a close friend, I began working for Vance International, a contract security company specializing in union strikes, and both VIP and asset protection. There, I found a company that appreciated my unique talents: situational awareness, attention to detail, organizational abilities, and keeping my own counsel. I loved the work, traveled a great deal, and made very good money. The camaraderie among the former military, Army Special Forces and police made me feel at home; my close friend was a former Navy Seal. We trusted each other with our lives, which were sometimes on the line during violent confrontations, and shared off-duty weeks hunting together on his farm in the mountains of Virginia.

The company promoted me regularly, giving me more and more responsibility, from documentary photography (recording evidence), and testifying in court cases, to shift supervisor, and the opportunity to work personal protection for a few executives and a couple of popular sports figures.

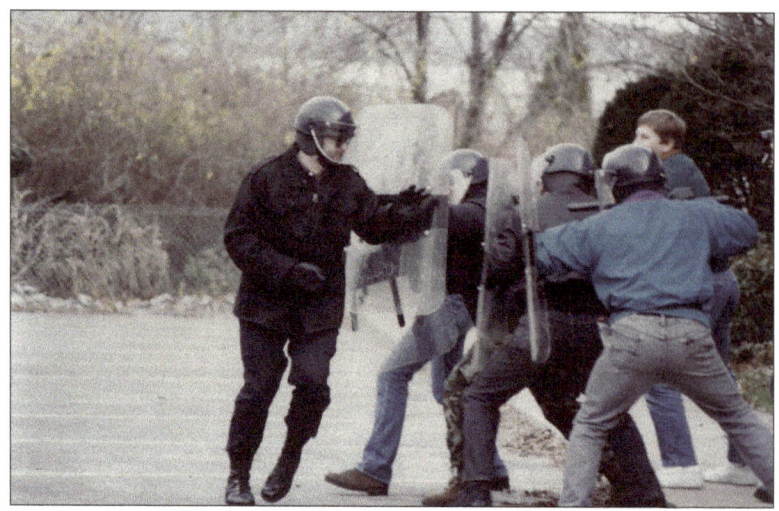
Riot Control Training

I eventually became an instructor and was responsible for organizing their recruiting schools, training the new employees in guard duty, evidence gathering including photo documentation, self-defense, and riot control. While teaching them tactics, we would beat on their helmets with batons and kick their riot shields to give them a sense of the realities that would soon face them. And I have to say, we got a real "kick" out of our work. Most of us were true adrenalin junkies. I had finally found a "home" for myself with a company that acknowledged my abilities and a group of men who had become like family to me.

One day in 1990, having just returned from a contract job, I was sitting in the small cabin I had purchased in the hills of Virginia reading the local newspaper. There was a personals ad from a lady seeking an outdoorsman for "life, love, and adventure." Well, that sounded interesting, so I sent her a letter and a photograph, figuring I might as well put all my cards on the table so there would be no misunderstanding. Two days later, I received a phone call; she wanted to meet for dinner. As I walked up to the back of the big blue van in the parking lot of The Little Chef restaurant and I looked into her eyes, I was head over heels in love. At our first meeting, it was as if our souls were created for one another. We closed down the restaurant, deep in conversation, while the waiters noisily stacked chairs on the adjoining tables and swept the floor under our feet. I'll let Alice tell you about the rest of our first date…

Alice: Lonely after a recently ended, humdrum relationship, I placed a personals advertisement in the Charlottesville Observer-Dispatch entitled "Outdoorsman Wanted." This was before the advent of internet dating. I am a professional wildlife and sporting dog artist, and I loved the Blue Ridge Mountains. I also loved hunting, fishing, canoeing, and hiking in them. My desire was for someone with whom I could share these experiences. With security in mind, I carefully made sure I did not list my phone or location, only a Post Office Box, and invited letters. I wanted to know how these men thought, from their writing, before I met them.

To my surprise, Russ was the only one who volunteered a photograph among the 17 letters I received. As I considered his photo, something almost audible came to my mind, and to this day the only explanation I have been able to consider was God, Whom I had rejected 4 years ago. "This man cares about his mother…" I later learned that this is an excellent gauge by which to measure a man's respect for women, including his wife.

When we met at the restaurant, Russ was so shy that he gripped the table with white knuckles. After I suggested we go to the salad bar, he said, "Go ahead. I'm a little nervous." I put my hand on his and said, "Don't be nervous. I'm just as scared of you as you are of me." By the end of the evening, almost four hours later, we were so deep in conversation, sharing our outdoor loves and experiences, that we didn't notice they were ready to close the restaurant!

So, we went and sat in his little red car and talked some more, about our principles and our lives. Then Russ asked me to come see where he lived, stating I could follow in my van. By this time I had thrown all security measures out of the proverbial window. "Oh no, its fine, I'll go with you." So we drove up to his "cabin", more accurately termed a shack. It had been the add-on to a mobile home but the mobile home was no longer there. He owned the five acres of land it stood on, and when we entered, I was impressed by his bookcase full of classics, and by the neatness of his housekeeping. We sat in the living room, Russ by the wood stove, and I across from him near the door, and continued our conversation for another hour at least.

Then, he got up, went to the door, closed it and threw the bolt. Alarms went off in my head! I've been too trusting! I'm going to die tonight! They'll find my body in a ditch somewhere! Mentally I planned to pick up the chair, break the window and escape if he came one step closer. Verbally, I said, "I am NOT comfortable with your locking that door!" Instead of doing or saying anything, he went back to his chair and wilted into it like a little lost puppy.

Since nothing threatening ensued, we eventually began our conversations again. And later I called my mother, who was visiting me from Australia, to tell her I would be really late coming home—but foolishly never gave her my location or Russ' phone number. I guess I had lost my mind in the intoxication of love, although I wouldn't admit it at the time. When I drove home another hour later, I tapped on my mother's guest room door and said, "Mom, I like him!" "Umm, yes," she mumbled. "Don't make up your mind too soon. Date some of those Charlottesville men before you decide." (Read: "Men with money.") "Yes, Mom," I said, and whispered a little prayer to the God I didn't believe in: O Lord, please help this to work out! Then I proceeded to call Russ the next day with an invitation to the Annual Outing of the Virginia Outdoor Writers' Association, of which I was a member. I'll tell you that story in a bit.

I didn't find out until weeks later that Russ had locked the door with the bolt because it didn't have a regular door handle, only a throw-bolt to keep it closed like a barn door. And he had been worried that the chill of the night was bothering me. He was so sure that he had ruined all prospects of dating me that he spent a miserable night, and was so delighted that I called the next morning. I also didn't find that out for a while!

We began spending a lot of outdoors time together. On our second date, we planned to go fishing on Greene Mountain Lake, where I lived in a nice rental house facing the Blue Ridge Mountains. It began to rain heavily, so we went into the walkout basement, where I had my framing and art storage area. We looked at a relief map of the nearby mountains, pointing out the trails we each had hiked, and found one near Luray that neither of us knew. All we did was look at each other, head for his car, and drive to the trailhead. On the way the rain had subsided to a light drizzle. Once on the main trail, we soon found a game trail leading up the side of the mountain. Of course we couldn't resist the challenge, so we climbed up through the forest, found a rock outcropping where we sat together and watched the sky clearing across the valley below. On the way back to the car, we saw a huge tree stump in the middle of the trail near its end. On impulse,

Russ jumped up on it, did a Peter Pan crow, and promised to "never grow up!" I did the same amid a gale of laughter. And we never did...

Our fourth date was a whitewater canoe trip down the James River which really cemented our budding relationship. We and all the veteran outdoor writers and authors, canoeing instructors, etc. put in at Scottsville, and headed downstream. Russ and I, novices at whitewater canoeing, put in last. As the group disappeared around the bend, we found ourselves stuck on top of a big mossy rock! Embarrassing to say the least, but fortunately not seen by anyone but ourselves, as we struggled to dislodge our canoe and get floating again. We laughed about it, got underway, and cast for a few smallmouth bass which we released. After catching up with the rest, we began to have advice shouted to us. They explained the difference in water flow among the rocks; one formation meaning "safe to go for it" and the other "watch out, underwater rock ahead!" We were really enjoying the new adventure, learning from everyone else, and making great headway. In fact, one of the canoes carrying two "old-timers" capsized, and lost all their expensive camera equipment; after they righted themselves, dripping wet and red-faced, we just kept paddling on. One man commented, "I still hear laughter coming from that canoe, so they must be doing OK!" The canoe instructor marveled that we were getting along so well; he never taught couples together since they usually ended up doing the "spouse stroke," bringing the paddle down sharply on the other's head in frustration and anger. Another said, "Maybe instead of premarital counseling, we should have premarital canoe trips to find out if people are compatible!" Wiser words were never said. We were working together in unison by this time. It had begun to rain, and Russ' glasses were fogging. So I, in the bow, would direct him as he power-paddled in the stern; I made the little swerves to avoid obstacles and let him know if any lay ahead. We were soon far forward of all the others. Alone on the broad and mighty James River, we enjoyed a group of otters who played with us. They would pop their heads up just in front of our canoe, look at us, roll and duck underwater, come up again downstream to wait for us, then do a repeat performance. As we went on in the drizzling rain, Russ and I planned our funerals, even before we spoke of a wedding: Have our bodies cremated, mix our ashes together, and be scattered here in the magnificent James River. This was a turning point in our lives, when we KNEW we made a great team. Never realizing that God was planning something for our futures, which needed teamwork. We had met on his birthday, September 28, 1990, and by early November, and my next art exhibit at the prestigious Easton Waterfowl Festival six weeks later, I was wearing his engagement ring. Despite what he says.

Then in 1991, eight months and six proposals later, we were married at Raven's Roost Overlook, milepost 11, on the Skyline Drive in Virginia.

And that was the beginning of the most incredible adventure imaginable. Immediately, God put in my heart a desire to accept my new responsibility as a husband and for our new life together. First, I asked Alice to join me in attending church, which she had repudiated along with belief in Christ. God used this decision to bring me closer to Him, and Alice back to Christ so we could walk together in faith. More about this later. Next, my position with Vance International required quite a bit of travel and being gone from home for several weeks to several months at a time.

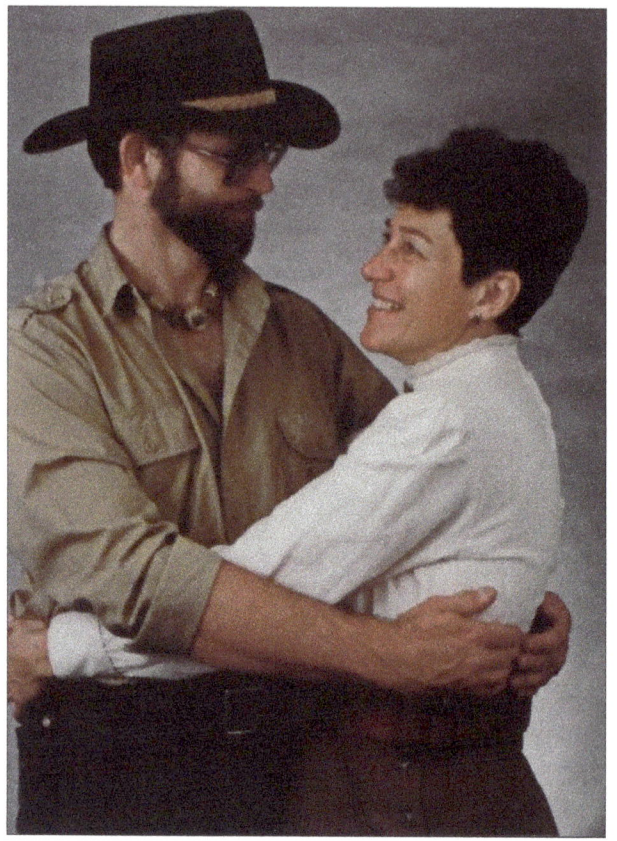

Russ and Alice's Engagement

I soon realized this could cause difficulties in any marriage. There is an old adage that says, "Absence makes the heart grow fonder." In my experience, a few days absence may make the heart grow fonder, but any extended absence will almost always give one too much time alone and encourage wandering thoughts. It became readily apparent to me something was wrong when I hadn't heard from Alice for a week, and I began to worry. I normally tried to write often and call whenever possible. We finally connected but we had allowed ourselves to become too busy and, not thinking clearly about it, put our relationship on the back burner. We realized almost too late we were beginning to drift apart. I had to decide what my priorities were, and I reluctantly resigned from the company to focus on building a new life together with Alice.

Alice: I am guilty of busy-ness. Always have been. We had tried to open a store, Buckhorn Art and Antiques, to develop a local business that would allow Russ to give up the long absences. The plan was to sell my artwork and his photography, which was transitioning from documentary to fine art, and a selection of antiques and collectibles. I was NOT cut out to spend long days sitting in a store, so in late 1994 I was shutting the business down in frustration. With some sense of failure—but also relief. And I was helping Russ' sister with a big bash—a surprise 50th Wedding Anniversary for his parents. Friends and guests from several states were invited, and all the planning and preparations for the party had to be done quickly and secretly. So yes, Russ got put on the back burner. I had excuses, didn't I? I was going to write him soon, when it was all over and I had all the Anniversary photos developed to send him. Then, when I found from our "long distance phone card" bill that he was making calls to other women we knew as friends, I was furious! I cancelled the card, stamped off in indignation to our pastor's wife to complain of Russ' borderline infidelity—and was taken aback when she looked at me sharply. "You promised to write to him, didn't you? And call him often?" Well, yes, but I was BUSY... "Did you do what you promised?" Well, no...but... "No excuses!" I was at fault for neglecting a very lonely man, far from home for months, in a lockdown situation, doing 12-hour shifts, responsible for a whole team of men under him in a possibly violent situation. After Becky opened my eyes, I realized how Russ had begun *to question MY sincerity and love—and had reached out to several friends we knew for human connection and harmless conversation. Thankfully, we were both closer to the Lord by now, and had made Him the head of our marriage. This was the only time we really came close to losing our relationship, and Christ helped us to heal it fairly quickly when Russ returned. This episode helped us with his decision.*

God was using Alice to redefine my relationship to Him, to reprioritize my life, to fill the empty longing in my heart, and to help me understand that the burden of guilt I had been carrying for so long was not of God. He had already forgiven me and I needed to forgive myself.

Chapter 3

Following Our Dream

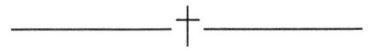

The first five years of our new life together were pretty typical. It had the ups and downs found in most young marriages, such as which way the slats on the window blinds faced, up or down, and who controls the temperature on the thermostat. But we resolutely struggled to unite these two lives into one unit. In 1994 I left my job with Vance International and joined Alice full-time in her art business. At that time she had already been a professional artist for 18 years and had a reputation as one of the finest wildlife and sporting dog painters in the U.S., with clients around the world.

We continued traveling to various wildlife art exhibitions and major dog shows where we could sell Alice's fine art paintings and limited edition prints. We made a good living and even bought a nice 33 acre property on a mountain in Southwest Virginia near the town of Galax, where we were determined to settle and build our future.

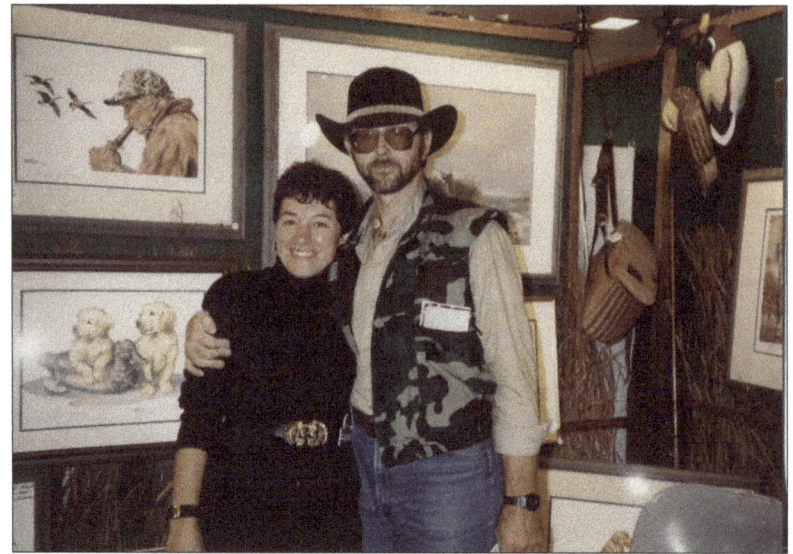

Alice's art, Easton Waterfowl Festival

It was the perfect place, nestled between vast forests and a wildlife management area with a stocked trout stream; and only 8 miles from Interstate 77 so we could reach our art markets easily. Turkey walked by our bedroom window each morning, ruffed grouse roosted in the oak trees, and deer came to drink from the creeks running down the mountain. Here, we intended to enjoy the outdoors and grow old together.

God had other plans for us.

Alice: Meanwhile, we began to live the life of our dreams. We had all the wildlife we could ask for at our doorstep. Trout in Crooked Creek Wildlife Management Area across the dirt road. Lady slippers, trillium, wild azaleas, and rhododendron in the mighty oak forest surrounding our house. Our home was well sited on a ridge between two small creeks, with a southern exposure toward North Carolina. Life was good!

We went to the little local newspaper, the "Galax Gazette" and offered our services as outdoor columnists. Our twice-monthly column, "Views from Buckhorn Ridge," was widely read in southwest Virginia and into North Carolina. In fact, when we went to a local Sportsmen's Show, some of the people said our column was the only reason they bought the paper! We made a great writing team, although, unknown to us, God was further forming us into a team for Him. Russ would gather facts, do interviews of outdoor notables, and put the information together. I would craft those facts into an interesting story, then Russ would edit for "too much fluff" and add his high quality photos. Our subjects ranged from nature to hunting to firearms legislation; everything from why God made vultures to the migration of Monarch butterflies to venison recipes to the philosophy of hunting. Our series on the timber industry received an award from the Forestry Industry of Virginia; one essay on hunting won Second Place in the state from the Outdoor Writers Association—just behind a column by a veteran writer in the prestigious Richmond newspaper! We thought this was to be our perfect life far into old age. But as Russ said, "God had other plans for us."

On our wedding day in 1991, we moved to Carroll County, Virginia. During this time God began to do a work in my heart and I started to feel a sense of responsibility as a new husband to be the spiritual leader in the family. After talking to Alice, we searched for a church home. Our first stop was at the First Baptist Church, Hillsville, and were immediately struck by the feeling of love and friendliness of the people. We had decided we would interview any prospective pastors to get a feel for their theology and friendliness. We still laugh about that after all these years. So, after meeting Pastor William Gunter and his wife Becky; and after attending services there and being impressed with his preaching, we decided to become members.

Alice: Prior to the time we met and married, I had rejected God and Christ, after being force-fed all my life in an abusive cult. My nature paintings soon convinced me that God was real, so I began asking Him the truth about Christ. It was at this point that Russ' quiet and deepening faith began to impact me. Once, he said, "Honey, I love you so much! I just regret we won't spend eternity together." That hit me. I continued seeking, telling others who showered me with Scripture, that I knew all that in my head. God needed to show me in my heart. And He did! One October morning in 1992, I woke before dawn, Russ sleeping at my side. I looked out the window through the branches of the bare oak trees, and there was the brilliant morning star glowing in the sky. Revelation 22:16b came to me, not in an audible voice, but as if someone had just spoken and I understood perfectly, "I am the Root and the Offspring of David, and the bright Morning Star." I knew Jesus was my Savior. I nudged Russ and said, "It's time to pray."

We began to work on our personal walk with the Lord and started daily devotions as a couple. God had a lot to teach us. Through studying God's word, I came to understand the importance of prayer in our lives. I learned that the Bible and prayer are the lines of communication with God. He was slowly, yet steadily becoming a part of our everyday lives. During this time we also made the decision that God must become the head of our marriage if it was to survive. And eventually, as I began to follow God's leading in my life; I also began to take on responsibilities in the church. I became the teacher of the College and Career Sunday School class with Alice as my co-teacher. It amazed me that the more I became involved with those young people as they sought God's direction in their lives, the more God used them to teach me.

I believe it was our fourth year as members of First Baptist Church in Hillsville, VA when the church family voted to start a second service which we named the Morning Glory Service. Soon after, I joined the worship team and helped plan the music for the service each week. As we went over song after song, I believe God began to speak to my heart through the music. One praise song became especially meaningful to me as the words penetrated deep into my heart.

It went like this:

> You are Lord of creation
> And Lord of my life,
> Lord of the land and the sea.
> You were Lord of the heavens
> Before there was time,
> And Lord of all lords You will be. [4]

As I sang that song, I started to listen to those words in a way I had never listened before, and they began to stir in my heart. And I felt God asking me, "Was Christ really Lord of my life?" And if He was; if I truly believed He was the Sovereign God, then I had to start living my life differently.

After that, the Morning Glory service took on a whole new meaning. Just about every Sunday, you could feel the presence of the Holy Spirit among us, and God was giving Pastor William some very powerful messages. During one such service

---

[4] We Bow Down, Twila Paris, 1984, Singspiration Music, Admin: Brentwood-Benson Music Publishing, Inc.

in April 1996, I was so strongly convicted by the Holy Spirit that I started crying. I knew that I had just had an encounter with God. And by the end of the service, when the invitation was given, I could stand it no longer. I went forward and told Pastor William that I wanted—NO, I MUST!—commit my life to God's service; to go wherever He wanted me to go, and do whatever He wanted me to do.

At the time I did not fully understand what it meant, and even though I have a better grasp now, to be perfectly honest, I was scared. I said, "God, I'm not all that smart, I have no training, and I have not been a very good person. How will I ever be able to serve you?" It was then that God gave us Proverbs 3:5-6 as our life verse. It says, "Trust in the Lord with all your heart, and lean not on your own understanding. In all your ways acknowledge Him, and He will make your paths straight."

It's true. It's real. And we continue to live it today.

Now, I had submitted my life to God, but not without reservation. I have to admit, I was afraid of what making a commitment to God really meant. It's one of those things that just sort of pops out of one's mouth, and you don't really think very deeply about the implication.

We fail to consider that when we give our lives over to God completely, life changes completely, and then not our will, but His will is done, and it is an unbelievable experience. It was not the one I had been seeking in my early life. This one was for real!

Alice: When Russ first began proposing "marriage" to me, I was terrified of the institution. My parents' relationship had been one constant power struggle, arguments and tears and misery. We children bore the brunt in physical abuse and sleepless nights. I did NOT want to get myself into another emotional prison like the one I had recently escaped. But, when I met his parents and saw their loving, laughing Christian relationship, I realized there was hope. Russ had grown up knowing what a good marriage was! I finally accepted his proposal but said, "NO submission stuff!" Submission of women in the Bible—erroneously translated by my father as "complete slavery"— had been used to beat me on the head all of my life. He smiled and agreed. But, when I saw Russ submit his life completely to the Lord on that day, submitting to Russ' leadership became possible for me.

Chapter 4

Putting Out the Fleece

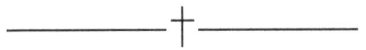

By the middle of 1996, God had placed me in a position as an announcer at a local Christian radio station known at the time as WBOB. It was Southern Gospel at its best. The General Manager, Debbie Epperson, had come up to me one day and said, "I like your voice. Would you like to work at my radio station?" It came as a bit of a surprise, considering I did not have any experience, but after a couple of weeks, I realized I enjoyed every minute of it. Debbie gave me *carte blanche*, letting me do anything I felt led to do as ministry, as long as I played the scheduled music, the advertisers' spots, and the Virginia Tech games. I began to read Scripture and short devotionals, make comments on the Gospel songs, and generally gave my on-air hours some personality. People began calling the station, asking for prayer and opening their hearts to me. They even asked if I were a pastor, which surprised me; that was the farthest thing from my mind. I thoroughly enjoyed my new ministry calling and put myself into it 100%. Yet, somehow I felt that God was leading me in another direction. It wasn't an audible voice, but a sense of restlessness and feeling there was so much more ahead of me.

One night during my shift at the radio station, I received a call from the Director of Missions of the New River Baptist Association, Bob Jackson. He asked if I would preach that Sunday evening during the service at the new Hispanic mission. I said, "But Bob, I'm not a preacher and it's almost midnight. I guess I could bring a devotional if you want, but I've never preached." He said, "No problem, whatever you can do would be a great help." So, I spent the rest of the night trying to throw together something for the service.

Alice: I always was interested in the many Hispanics that began flooding into our country in search of a better life. After picking up some rudimentary Spanish, I was happy to hear of the new Mission our Association had begun in Galax. Russ consented to my volunteering, but said he would drive me there, since it was in a questionable part of town and the service ended after dark on Sunday nights. Because of his wonderful singing voice, he was "volunteered" to be Music Leader. God must have smiled! Russ is not good with languages, and didn't know more than two words of Spanish. So, he chose hymns and Gospel songs with melodies he knew, and we found the Hispanic lyrics for them. I taught him basic pronunciation, and all was fine. Well, just a few smiles and chuckles now and then. But the people, refugees from poverty in their own countries of Mexico, El Salvador, Guatemala, and more, were delighted to have a place to worship God in their own language. It gave them a sense of community far from all they had known.

We soon heard a rumor of a renegade Hispanic bakery in a trailer park; after knocking on the door, a young boy poked his head out. We convinced him we were not the INS, but were looking for bakery products. After entering the flour-dusted living room filled with ovens, we were intoxicated with the aroma of wonderful pastries. Loading our bags with gorditos and pan dulces, we became regular customers, providing after-service snacks at the Hispanic Mission. I still miss that delicious food!

Well, the service seemed to go pretty well. The interpreter took up a lot of the time, and the congregation only laughed twice. I have to say I was glad when it was over. After a few more times of this, another night around midnight, as usual, Bob called and said he had to be at another church that Sunday and needed me to fill in again. And as usual, I said "fine." But then he said, "Oh, by the way, this time I need you to preach at Sharon Springs Baptist Church." "Church!" I said. "Wait a minute, that's a real church. I don't preach, I just do devotionals." Bob said, "Just do your best. They will understand." Good grief. How did this ever happen? I never, ever thought I would do something like this. So anyway, I took one of my devotionals and expanded on it to fill up almost thirty minutes and prayed for the best.

We arrived a bit early and took a seat on the front pew waiting for the service to begin. In hobbled the pastor. He had fallen off his roof while doing some repairs, but still came for the service with a cast up to his hip and crutches. He came over and plunked down beside me, looked me in the eye and said, "What version of the Bible are you preaching from?" Good grief! I should have known. I had begun using the NIV a couple of years earlier and never considered it might be a problem. I had stumbled into a "King James Only" church. I explained that I had developed the message around scripture verses from the NIV, and even had it all typed out. He said, "I was afraid of that. Oh well, go ahead, I'll just put the fires out after you're gone." Talk about a confidence builder, now I was approaching panic.

Anyway, I stood up, gave the message and afterward everyone told me how well I did. I even got a couple of "Amens" while I was speaking. Needless to say, I was relieved. After we left and were heading down the road, Alice turned to me and said, "Maybe God is calling you to preach." I went ballistic. "Oh NO, I don't preach, I only do devotionals!" But from that moment on, I could not get it out of my mind. Hiding behind the radio microphone had bolstered my confidence, but I still avoided standing in front of people to speak, unless there was no way out.

One day at the radio station, I read an article in *The Religious Broadcaster's Magazine* about radio as a ministry. Following the article was a list of colleges that offered a degree in Christian Broadcasting. That sounded interesting. It occurred to me that if this was the ministry God had for me, then I needed to get some training to be more effective on the radio. So, in 1997, I was off to Toccoa Falls College in Toccoa, Georgia.

Alice: You have to understand that WBOB Radio was using vintage equipment. Most broadcast stations by that time were almost totally computerized. For instance, on Saturdays, Russ came in early, used a broomstick to push the huge overhead horseshoe switch "On" to power the transmitter tubes. Yes, tubes! Then he had to wait for an hour for them to warm up before going on the air. When he got to Toccoa Falls College, the equipment he had been using was in their Radio Museum. Yes, further education was a dire necessity if he were to continue.

And I guess I have to tell another story of how God works! We had just moved from our dream home on the mountain, to live near Galax so Russ could be close to his radio ministry. When he told me of his vision to get a degree in Christian Broadcasting, I sighed. Not moving again! So, I began to write a list of requirements that would have to be met before we could do this—certain that they would never materialize, and I would be safe in our current house.

First, we had just gotten completely debt-free after selling our mountain home. So, I stipulated that Russ would have to get a job to pay for his tuition, and not take out student loans. And of course I would have to get a job—never having had a "real" one before. I had worked for my father for no pay for years, then had my own art and antique business ever since. So, I had no real world work experience. The job I needed would have to pay $1200 per month take-home at minimum, and even then, we would have to rent a house at less than $300 per month. Ha! Never happen! Add to this that Russ did not have his acceptance to TFC finalized. All this in late December 1996. Smugly, I didn't think the risk of moving again was very high. I forgot that God has His own plans—but my fleece was out. (See Judges 6:37)

Russ, bent on his dream, called TFC and his Application Counsellor said the official acceptance letter was on its way. Then he called their WRAF flagship radio station to inquire about a part-time job to help pay tuition. They replied that was not likely, since many Broadcasting students did their practicum there, but "send down a demo tape anyway." Russ sighed and said he needed to find his wife a job, too. The lady asked what I did; he replied professional artist. That opened the floodgates. "Well, there's a big furniture manufacturer here in Toccoa, Habersham Plantation, which makes nationally-known art furniture. They're always hiring staff artists. Let her call them." Uh-oh. My fleece was getting a little dampness on it.

I called them and sent a portfolio. They scheduled an interview for January 17, 1997, my birthday. TFC was 5 hours away so I decided to spend 2 days, scope out the college and housing *situation as well. I nervously went to my first job interview at 54 years old, and after questioning me, they ushered me out the door with "We'll call you." I was certain that meant "no!" I asked them for directions to the college and met with the Dean of Married Students, explaining our needs for jobs and housing. He gave me a listing of landlords and other advice. Meanwhile, the phone rang and he handed it to me. I assumed it was Russ inquiring about the job interview—but it was Habersham, telling me I had the job! It paid $500 per week during my training period copying paintings on armoires, tables, etc. and I was expected to do at least that much afterword on piecework. This would be a new experience for me! Hmmm, that translated to taking home $1200 per month. Where did I hear this before?*

So I went back to the motel and began to call realtors listed in the newspaper. "$300 per month? Hahaha." Then I began to call landlords from the TFC list. Many said just go, find the hidden key and look at the house. That didn't work out too well. Then I called Tom Dooley, a former Olympic runner, who had many rental homes specifically for students and elderly. Not fancy, but renovated to functional. He had 2 homes available at $250 and $275 per month. The best house was on the main road to the college and only a quarter mile from my work. And he even mowed the grass since he had a few storage units on the rear of the property. I called Russ and said it's time to rent the U-Haul. God had drenched my fleece and it was wringing wet. I never tried that again! By the way, we ended up going to Tom's church, Grace Baptist, which later played a prominent part in our future ministry.

Now, remember, by then I was almost 49 years old. So going to college was an adventure in itself. And then, instead of continuing to pursue a degree in communications that I thought

God wanted me to do, He made an end run around me and called me into pastoral ministries. That was a real shocker, not only to me, but to my friends and family that had known me for most of my very turbulent life, and had a ring-side seat.

Alice: One of our friends from Zimbabwe, also attending TFC, was having dinner with us at our little rental home. Derek asked Russ what his major was. Derek then leaned over the back of our sofa, slapped it repeatedly while laughing aloud. "Russ is going to be a pastor!!! Ah hahaha!"

At that point, I began preaching and holding Bible studies at Victory Home, a drug and alcohol rehabilitation center in Northeast Georgia. The men there found they could not hoodwink me, and that I understood their lives only too well. They often tested me and found that I was the real thing, and most of all, God was the real thing. He had changed my life completely. And He could do the same for them.

Chapter 5

Time to Pack Your Bags—Again

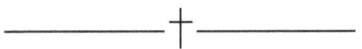

During a Missions Conference in February of 1998, I was in the gym at Toccoa Falls College looking at the ministry displays set up by several different mission organizations. The college held the Conference every year as an opportunity for students to see what these organizations offered for mission service around the world, and to get some sense of where God might be leading them into short-term ministry during the following summer. I was impressed by all the huge, professional displays, glossy color photos, and blinking lights on world maps. Then, way back in the corner of the gym was a tiny, inconsequential card table with a few small images. An older couple was talking to students about a radio ministry called "Voice for Christ" in Nenana, Alaska, way up in the Interior.

After talking to them for a few minutes I was so excited about what I heard that I quickly drove home. Running into the house, I shouted to Alice, "Honey! You need to see something!"

Alice: I've come to learn this phrase means "time to pack my bags!"

So, off to the college campus we went. After looking at the pictures on the display board, Alice turned to me and said, "I've seen that bridge before! I've been there!" And so she had. Back in 1987, she had made a trip with a professional photographer friend who wanted company on the excursion and help with the expenses. Marvina Munch was not much of an outdoors woman, but she had an adventurous spirit. It was Alice's first experience in the North Country outside the lower 48, but unknown to her at the time, it was not to be her last.

After much prayer and a few phone calls to the ministry, we made the decision to spend the next summer serving as short-term missionaries in Nenana. It was a small radio station situated in the interior of Alaska. KIAM was founded by Bob and Dee Eldridge and ministered to a vast wilderness without churches or missionaries, via a couple of radio translators throughout the "bush" of central Alaska. We had an awesome time and we were blessed greatly by the experience, as well as getting to know two great people who committed their lives to broadcasting the gospel throughout Alaska.

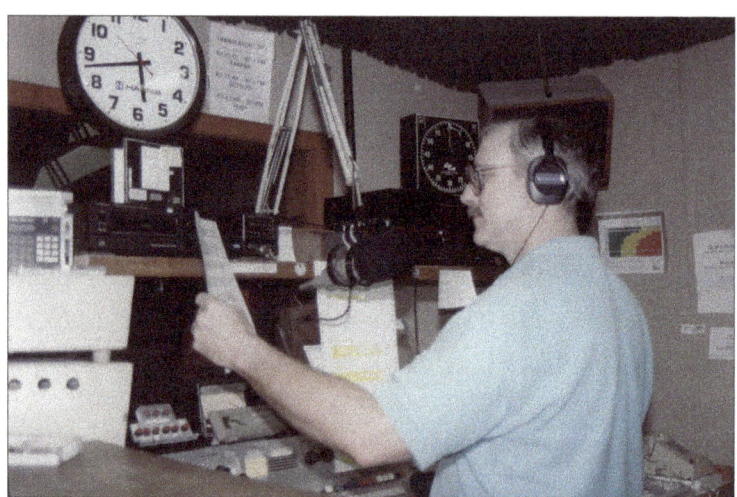

Russ On-Air, KIAM Radio

We discovered that the Alaskan Interior has a totally different culture and geography than I had ever experienced. Yes, Fairbanks, where we flew in, is a pretty typical American city with lower temperatures in winter, but the rest of the vast area is completely foreign in many ways.

Our first impressions were of forests that began at the city limits, moose wandering the power line cuts and snow-capped mountains on every horizon. Another thing that will stay with us forever is the scent of spruce trees in the cool, clean air.

The village of Nenana was on the Parks Highway, one of the few paved roads in the entire state. At the intersection of the Parks and the Tanana River, it was a hub of transportation and freight for thousands of square miles of wilderness. Even though Nenana was small in population, it was in a key location wisely chosen for the KIAM radio ministry.

One myth that was soon dispelled was the fantasy of rugged log cabins for homes. There were a few, but there were also typical American ranch houses, split-levels, and many old mobile homes with wannigans (ramshackle plywood additions) attached, sometimes covered with ugly spray foam insulation. The yards were often filled with rusting 55-gallon drums, broken snow machines, firewood in various stages of preparation, and occasionally "yellow iron" (bulldozers etc.) and aircraft parts. The philosophy was "ya never know when it might come in handy." What was the use of tidying up when the few months of summer were spent in preparing for the long winters? All the junk was soon covered with snow anyway. It became obvious this was a land where survival was a daily challenge. That summer changed us forever. We reluctantly flew back to Georgia and school in the fall.

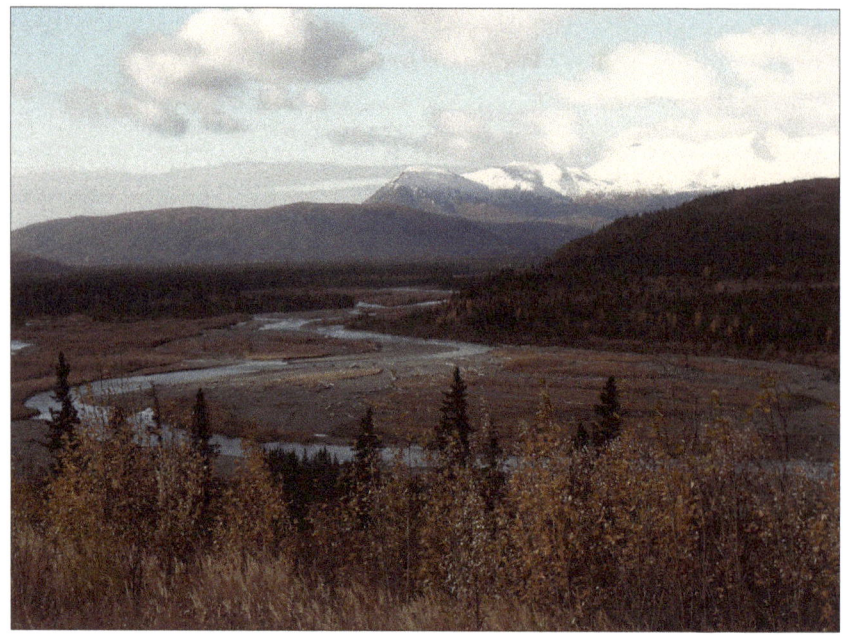

The Alaskan Interior

The school year went by swiftly. And once again we were considering where we might take our next summer mission trip. During the school year Bob Eldridge kept calling us to come back. I told him we hadn't made a decision yet but would be in prayer about it. Alice and I decided we would try other mission opportunities because we didn't want to return to Alaska based on a purely emotional experience. Let's face it. Alaska is one of the last great frontiers in North America. It's sparsely populated and cold, but a majestic wilderness. Just our cup of tea.

We prayed regularly and contacted several other possible summer mission organizations and nothing materialized. Alice and I had decided some time ago that we always ask God's guidance before making any decisions. Our prayer was that if God opened the door that is the direction we would go. And if the door was closed we believed it was not in God's will.

Finally, we gave in and I called Bob to let him know we would be coming back that summer.

We ended up serving two summers with Bob and Dee in Nenana. It was a wonderful experience, and a time of personal and spiritual growth for us both, and only fired up my desire to serve God in areas most others were not going to or being effective for whatever reason. But two "divine appointments" arranged by the Lord happened that second summer that began to add clarity to our future. Every morning during the second trip, Alice would take her daily walk around the village. She eventually became known as the "woman who walks." On one of those walks she met Margaret Sanders, the director of the Senior Center. She became fast friends with Alice and invited us to come for lunch at the center 3 days a week. She was to become our "person of peace" and introduce us to village life.

The second "divine appointment" was when Alice was supposed to be home making me lunch while I was working my "on air" shift.

Alice: It was the second summer that we had a "Macedonian Call" experience. (Acts 16:9-10) I was the Station Receptionist each morning, so headed across to the old mobile home where we stayed, to make lunch for Russ when he got off his shift. Ahhh, if you only knew me.... In crossing the gravel street, I noticed a Yard Sale a few blocks up. It would only take a few minutes to check it out. Yeah, right. I saw a nice nylon jacket, picked it up while the Native lady came out of the log cabin to sell it to me. I mentioned that the sleeves were dirty, and besides we were at the Radio Station and were leaving in a week. She was not daunted. "Radio Station! I'm a believer! My grandchildren are believers! Come on, I'll wash it for you!" Then, the clincher. "My son in Fairbanks is an alcoholic and he's threatening suicide. I've been trying to find a pastor to pray with me, but no one answers their phones." So, of course I blurted out, "I'll pray with you! I'm so sorry you can't locate even one pastor. My husband and I have been wondering if this village needs a new church really involved with its people." So, for the next hour we prayed. And prayed. And Florida Gierke prayed, "O Lord, please bring Russ and Alice to start a new church here!" So I eventually made my way back to the mobile home—and a hungry Russ—with the strange feeling that we had just been called by God.

Upon returning to Toccoa at the end of the summer of 1999, we were confident that Alaska was in our future. But the first of many health concerns suddenly arose. I had been strong, healthy and active all of my life, despite abusing my body terribly in my roaming years. Just when Alice and I felt we had a goal to focus on, the evil one attacked. I'll let Alice tell the story from her perspective.

Alice: We had returned from Alaska with dreams of the future forming in our minds. Alaska! The Last Frontier! Exciting adventure lay ahead. I settled back into my job at Habersham, whose Christian owner, Matt Eddy, graciously allowed me six weeks off each summer for our mission trips. When I came home from work a few days later, Russ began reading aloud to me from Frank Peretti's "Piercing the Darkness." Just as he got to a passage about a conflict between mighty angels and other spiritual beings, he put his hand to his chest. I asked what was happening. He said, "Oh, it goes away..." "WHAT goes away?" "Oh, a little twinge." "How long has this been going on?" "Oh, maybe three or four days. But it goes away..."

But he did not take his hand away, so I asked if it were worse today. He admitted it was. I then asked if the pain were going down his left arm. Yes, it was. I stood up, grabbed the keys, and said, "We ARE going to the Emergency Room!" He assented; I think he too was beginning to get worried.

The small hospital in Toccoa could find nothing wrong with his EKG, but the wise elderly doctor said that something must be amiss, since the pain subsided immediately with a nitroglycerin patch. He sent us to Athens Regional Heart Hospital, where they did an angiogram. Sure enough, the "widow-maker" (right descending anterior artery of the heart) was 60% blocked; so a stent was inserted as Russ watched on the TV monitor. All went well.

The next morning a nurse came in to remove the shunt from his femoral artery; all did not go well this time. Apparently the pre-op dose of Plavix blood thinner had been too much for Russ' body. The site began to bleed. And bleed. And bleed.

The nurse attempted pressure, but it didn't work. He nervously called in other nurses, who attempted to halt the hemorrhage. They couldn't. I watched numbly while they sopped up blood with huge handfuls of gauze; my husband's blood, lots of it. I must have turned grey because they asked me to step out of the room. As I did, I saw them bring in a plastic "bridge" with a ball on each end to place on his groin arteries; pass a strap under him to secure it; then pump it up with air to bring extreme pressure on the vessels. The bleeding finally subsided but I heard them say his blood pressure was now 50-something over 39…

Meanwhile, I was leaning against the wall in the hallway, praying hard. I turned as they rushed Russ out of the room on a gurney, heading hastily for ICU. I reached over and touched *his head as they rushed by, thinking this may be the last time I see him alive.*

As they were rushing me down the hall, I asked the nurse by my head if there was anything I could do. "Just keep breathing!" She said. "I can do that," I said. Then she leaned over and asked if there was anything I wanted her to tell my wife. I knew what that meant! This was serious.

Alice: I found my way to the ICU waiting room. And continued in prayer. I asked the Lord to heal Russ, but if it wasn't His will, to help me deal with it. At that moment, I gave Russ completely to the Lord; he was no longer mine, but a vessel of God.

They sent in a New Age "chaplain", but I didn't need her. I needed the Lord—and Russ. After several interminable hours, they let me see him. He was conscious, resting quietly, but the last huge wad of gauze, full of dried blood, was still between his legs. They apparently didn't want to disturb the wound again. By that time, Pastor Joel from Grace Baptist Church had arrived; and the attending nurse asked Russ if there was anything he wanted. Yes, of course! Some ice cream! She brought two containers of ice cream which he ate with gusto. Russ spent a few more days in the hospital to make sure all was well. The nurse who initially tried to remove the shunt came in daily to visit with him, obviously relieved Russ hadn't died.

The first Sunday we returned to church, Pastor Joel welcomed us back from the pulpit, then told the whole congregation something that amused him. Here was a man who had to have a stent due to heart blockage from fats; who almost died from the procedure; and the first thing he asked for in ICU was ice cream! Worse yet, the nurse gave him not only one serving, but two! We all laughed...it was good to be alive.

God had spared me, and I knew He had a purpose for us. But first I had something to learn. As I spoke in gratitude to God during my devotional time He gave me another verse to keep in my heart, "For to me, to live is Christ and to die is gain." (Philippians 1:21)

I believe that God wanted me to understand that death is a great loss only to a worldly person, because he loses all his earthly comforts and all his hopes; but to a true believer it is a gain. "To live is Christ" means that we are to pursue the knowledge of Christ. Not just a set of facts about Christ, but Christ Himself. And that we are to be willing to give up everything that prevents us from having Christ. Christ is our focus, our goal, and our chief desire. And everything that we do, we do for Christ's glory.

From that moment on, it was like riding a whirlwind. Toccoa Falls College decided to raise their tuition, so we moved to Kansas City, MO, where I enrolled at Midwestern Baptist Theological Seminary. They had a plan through the North American Mission Board called the Nehemiah Project, a church planting program under the supervision of an extremely capable professor, Director of Missions, and a bit of a renegade named Carrol Fowler. We had traveled to the Midwestern campus to spend three days exploring the seminary and the possibility of attending school there. Making my way across the parking lot to where we were staying, I saw this big, burly man walking right up to me, who then threw his arm around my shoulders and said, "You must be Russ. Your wife told my wife you were interested in going to Alaska. Well son, I can help you with that!" And I'm thinking, "Who is this guy anyway?" I soon found out.

Chapter 6

The Next Great Adventure

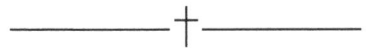

I began classes at Midwestern the following spring semester and had the opportunity and privilege of getting to know Carroll, not only as a very effective church planting professor, but as a friend and mentor. He took Alice and me under his wing and taught us to "think outside the box" of accepted church tradition, and sent us back to Nenana, Alaska the next summer with ten weeks of financial support.

We were given the task of doing a demographic survey, and gauging the need for a new church in this community of 450 residents. When we arrived we were politely told that if there was a need for a new church the "establishment" in Fairbanks would have started a work there already. And besides, it would be at least five years to get anywhere in this "hardened" area. But God continued to remind us to, "Trust in the Lord with all your heart…"

Alice and I began our assessment by making the rounds and introducing ourselves and giving each home a small gift. We gave them a light bulb, to light their home, and a New Testament to give light for their souls. The wife of the Native chief, Katherine Demientieff, remarked, "This is strange. You are the newcomers to the village, and you are giving *us* gifts?" The gossip flew; the "Alaska grapevine" is one of the fastest news networks known to man. Grace Baptist Church from Toccoa, GA heard of our venture, and brought a mission team, half teenagers and half adults, to help us for a week. We went in pairs around the village, which was 40% Native Athabascan and 60% Anglo, visiting each home, and asking them what they would like to see in a new church, and presenting the Gospel.

Grace Baptist volunteered to help us with a public meeting in the Community Center to introduce the concept of a new church, and offered to pay for a catered meal. Scheduled for 6PM Saturday, July 1st, we soon realized the date was probably a big mistake. Many of the villagers would travel to the city of Fairbanks for July 4th festivities, a major celebration in Alaska. Most native people would be traveling down to the village of Tanana, at the confluence of our Tanana River and the Yukon, for a huge Memorial Potlatch for a native leader who had died in a plane crash. Saturday arrived, and by the 6 o'clock starting time our Team was virtually alone in the Community Center. Two teen boys sat at the rear of the huge room, rocking their chairs back against the wall, waiting for that catered meal to show up. I decided we needed the Lord to intervene; so Pastor Joel of Grace Baptist, all the men on the Team, and myself went into the little kitchen, closed the door and began to pray.

By the time we emerged, the women, who were waiting to register attendees at the door, had run out of chairs to seat the crowd! One person had lost count at 129, out of a village of 450. Over 25% of the population had come! The teens did a powerful mime skit depicting Christ overcoming the devil; people stood on chairs to watch. Phil Marsten from Toccoa sang a solo he had written. Pastor Joel preached a powerful message, with the familiar illustration of a train bridge watchman who saw his little son climbing into the works of the lift bridge; as the passenger train approached, the man had to choose between killing his own son, or letting hundreds of people die. He chose to sacrifice his son…as God did for us. Just then, as the Pastor was telling this story, the train going past the village blew its whistle loud and clear! Now, you have to understand that there is only one railroad in all of Alaska, and it came through our village. For this to happen at that precise moment was the hand of God. And it impacted the crowd deeply!

We had 33 professions of faith that night. After the service, Pastor Joel asked me what I had planned for the church service the next day. The question stopped me in my tracks because I had not yet thought that far ahead. Within four weeks of stepping off the plane in Fairbanks, God had planted a new church! God had prepared the soil and we were willing to sow the seeds.

Praise His Name!

The Athabascan matriarch of the village, Mary Demientieff, commented, "I never in my life seen anything like this!" Neither had we! Nor the village! So many people showed up that night that our team was not able to eat any of the delicious dinner. We went to our cabins late that night, tired, amazed, and excited!

Alice: But it was not yet over. Alaska is a place of spiritual darkness, as well as physical darkness in the long winters. Alcohol and drugs are rampant, suicide common, and demon worship is a way of placating the evil spirits at work there. After the excitement of seeing a new church born, we experienced spiritual warfare within a few hours. Russ awoke about 1AM, sweating profusely. He felt so weak he could not raise up on his elbow for me to give him a drink of water. Something was oppressing him, and he had no strength to fight it. I ran down the street to the Bed and Breakfast where the Mission Team was staying. Concerned that I would be awakening everyone from deep sleep, I was surprised to see the lights blazing. I hurried in, and said, "Something is very wrong with Russ! We need someone to come!" The Team was up, and several of the teen girls appeared shaken and somber. They had been having terrible nightmares of dark shapes coming to capture them, and awakened everyone with their screams. Phil and Sandy Marsten hurried back with me to our one-room cabin, and prayed fervently over Russ. He felt a great weight lifting off him, and the sweating subsided. Soon he was able to fall asleep in peace. Phil and Sandy left, and we all talked about our common experiences the next day. Satan is not happy when you invade his territory, but "…the one who is in you is greater than the one who is in the world." (1 John 4:4) God had planted a new church, and He would watch over it.

The next week, we held a Baptism Service. Four of the people who had accepted Christ at the Community Meeting wanted to follow in obedience to Christ's command, so the Bed and Breakfast owned by Gayle and Charlie Stevens graciously allowed us to use their small indoor pool. A fifth candidate for baptism was my own wife. What a blessing and a privilege!

Alice: During my growing years, everything was decided for me and forced upon me. At fourteen, I was baptized. But after coming to the Lord on my own, after I married Russ, I felt I also needed to be baptized by my own choice. And who better to do the ceremony than my own husband, who was following the Lord with all his heart? I will admit that as he lowered me into the pool, my feet flew up, floating, and he almost lost me into the water. Ah, well…we both survived!

Since the Community Center did not allow regular religious meetings, I began to hold services under a pavilion between the railroad and the Tanana River. Besides the mosquitos which tortured us (Alaska has 27 varieties, all fierce and hungry), the train would often interrupt my Sunday sermons. Then we met in our tiny one-room rental cabin, which was filled to bursting. Finally as our time came to an end for the summer, the church moved into the homes of various members, and it was time to return to Midwestern Seminary and report on our progress.

Alice: Opposition sometimes comes from unexpected places. The Alaska Baptist Convention, which provided part of our summer funding, received a "complaint" from persons in Fairbanks that "baptisms were going on in Nenana and they should check it out." Dave Baldwin, formerly from Fairbanks and now in the State office, sent Ken and Barbie (Yes, those were really their names) up to Nenana see what was happening. They stepped into our tiny cabin and apologized for the "complaint" they were investigating, stating that there should have been rejoicing in those quarters instead. Russ explained why we were here, what God had done, and also assured them that he was officially licensed to the ministry. Ken then smiled and asked if they could help us in any way; we really needed assistance with our huge phone bill, since it was the old days of long-distance dial-up internet. They gladly did so, and went back to report to Dave and the Alaska Baptists that God had birthed a new church in Nenana, and gave us their blessings!

It was now August and time to make a major decision in our life. Go back and finish my last year and one half of seminary, leaving this newly birthed church on its own, or leave seminary and continue the work that God so obviously had ordained here in the village of Nenana, Alaska. After a couple of weeks of prayer and discussion, we headed back to Midwestern where I explained what had happened, received a refund of my next semester's tuition, and was sent off with prayer and well wishes from all our professors and friends. Carroll Fowler, of course, was smiling. He knew his teaching would be effective. And I believe he is still smiling today. On June 21, 2004, Carroll quietly went home to be with his Lord during routine knee replacement surgery. He was a great friend and mentor, and a prolific church planter. He loved the Lord and he loved the church. We will never forget the lessons we learned from his decades of experience.

We first went to see a few churches, including Grace Baptist, to report on what the Lord had done; Tom Dooley loaned us a camper van to drive up the Alcan Highway, towing a 9x12 U-Haul trailer with our few worldly possessions, mostly my books. We were promised a fully furnished older mobile home to rent in the middle of the village where we would also be holding church. So, off we went on another great adventure— God's, so different from my early years. We headed off across the U.S. and up into Canada where I saw my first Northern Lights in Edmonton, Alberta. The next stretch of our drive took us through British Columbia and over the Continental Divide, where we saw Stone sheep and caribou crossing the road; stopping on the summit of Steamboat Mountain, where we rested ourselves and the weary van. We spent a short time looking out across hundreds of miles of wilderness; then drove on into Whitehorse, Yukon Territory where we stayed for a day or two and went to the public library to check our e-mail.

Alice: I almost had a heart attack. We were 4000 miles from our starting point, and still had 1000 miles to our destination—but the mobile home we had been promised was not available. The family who lived in it had nowhere else to go. There was another one, several miles out of town deep in the forest along the railroad, but how could we hold church out there? Who would come? Besides, we had sold almost all our furniture and even our dishes! What would we do? As Russ keeps saying, "Trust in the Lord…"

We jolted wearily onward over the frost heaves and potholes into Alaska, past Tok and Delta Junction, on through Fairbanks, and down to Nenana, arriving there on my birthday, September 28. It was snowing as we unpacked our U-Haul in a shed, then we went on down the road to our new home. We lived in that old, cold mobile home for the next three wintery months, holding church in the village at members' homes, and wondering what had happened to all our well-laid plans.

Alice: Since we did not have much missionary support, I took a job at the sole gas station/ convenience store in Nenana, the "A-Frame." It gave us some cash, plus helped me to get to know many of the villagers. Dave and Nancy Shaw were great employers, and their son Aaron, who has Down syndrome, was my cheerful instructor. He really knew how to run the store!

Meanwhile, knowing Tom Dooley was soon flying up from Georgia to pick up his van camper, we decided to look for a used vehicle in Fairbanks. We tried many venues, then someone suggested "The Lemon Lot" at Ft. Wainwright, the army base. Servicemen, transferring out to their next duty station, would put their vehicles up for sale here, with phone numbers in the windows. We called several, and finally one man showed up and let us try out his Grand Caravan. We liked it, and Russ explained that we needed to contact a church who had promised to help us with the purchase. The man learned we were planting a new church in Nenana, so as I was test-driving the car around the lot, he was on the phone. As I returned, he took the keys and handed them to Russ. "Drive it home," he said. "It's yours!" God always provides!

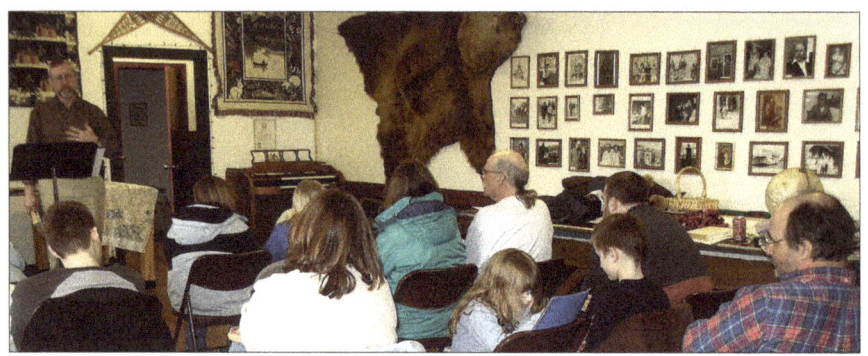

Russ Preaching

One day in January, I saw a "Moving Sale" posted on the bulletin board in the store. I knew where the rental house was, and I knew that Margaret Sanders' son was the absentee owner. I called the tenants and asked if the house was up for rent, then I asked them to tell Margaret that we definitely WANTED it! It was in town, large enough to hold us and have the church meet there. So, for the next several years, this old log home was Nenana Community Church as well as our home. The great room was the sanctuary. The Arctic entry (mud room) was the tweens' Sunday school; our master bedroom the children's class (they loved bouncing on the bed); the many teenagers had theirs in the great room; and the adults squeezed into the second bedroom, which was Russ' office. It was also the place where the many nursing mothers fed their infants during service. On Easter, we had 50 people attending, sitting on folding chairs; children sat on a sleeping bag on the floor near the pulpit. God was blessing the ministry!

Nenana Community Church continued to grow and impact the village of Nenana, and through a 3-day summer basketball camp each year we were able to influence the youth for Christ all over the state of Alaska. You have to understand that young people in Alaska not only play basketball, they eat, sleep and dream it. Randy and Jamie of *Crossfire Ministries*, former UNC basketball players, came every August to coach and hone basketball skills. Between sessions, they would present the Gospel of Jesus Christ. We had counsellors ready to work with individual young people who wanted to know more. They were often mission team members, such as one group from Webber Memorial Baptist Church in Chesterfield, VA, where our first pastor, William Gunter, was now in ministry. He and Becky saw the fruits of his mentoring all those years ago in what God was doing in faraway Alaska. God has given us many long term friends who have been with us since the beginning of our walk with Him!

Another amazing thing happened. The public school was allowing us to use their facilities for the camp. By the third year, they insisted on being listed as a sponsor in our advertising. The effectiveness of the event was obvious and we were delighted that they wanted to openly partner with what the Lord was doing through the Church.

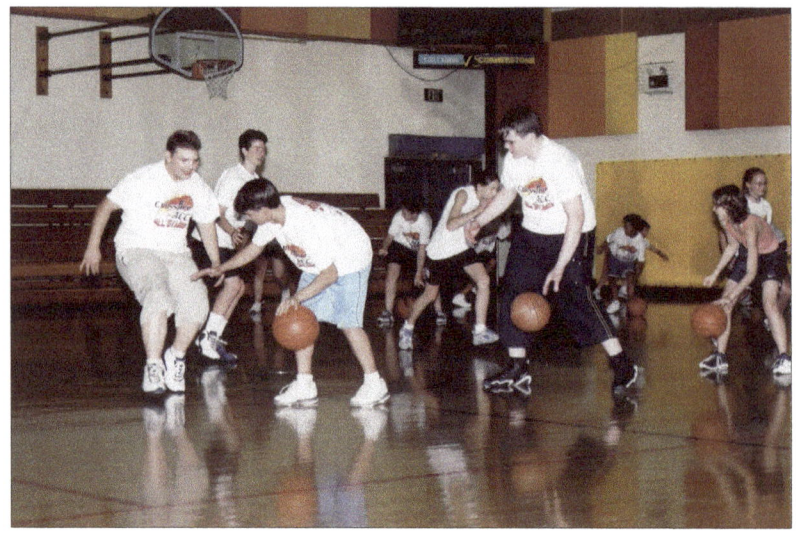

Crossfire Basketball Drills

During one of these camps, our ladies' coordinator, Ramona Chrisman, doubted we could feed all the young people on our tiny budget. We had over 60 youth housed in the Student Living Center besides mission team members, using their cafeteria for meals, and the school gymnasium for the coaching. She and Alice began buying food and planning menus, then God began to work. A food distributor in Fairbanks showered us with a huge donation of bread products and chips. Others followed suit. At the end of the event, we had food left over, almost twelve baskets full!

Students flocked to the Camp from all over Alaska, from near Anchorage 6 hours to the south, to Barrow on the Arctic Ocean, a span of over 700 miles. Native boys from remote villages were brought 100 miles up the Tanana River in their family's flat bottomed boats and dropped off on the shore. Two Inuit boys from Barrow attended one year. During a jam session one evening in the dorms, they gave their lives to Christ, then requested prayer for their alcoholic parents.

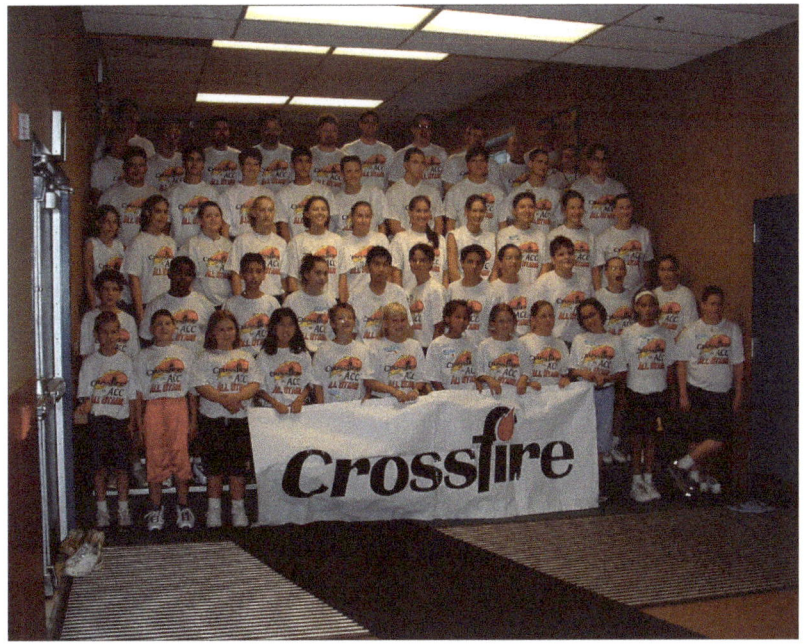

Kids, Crossfire Coaches and Mission Team

The finale of the camp each year was a demonstration of the newly acquired skills of their children in front of all the parents, followed by an entertaining Gospel presentation by Jamie and Randy using basketballs. In answer to prayer, the parents of those two Inuit boys gave their lives to Christ. Later, they gave the coaches and myself each a piece of whale baleen inscribed with Scripture verses. Mine is still hanging over my desk, a deeply treasured reminder of God's faithfulness and power to change lives. God does answer prayer!

Alice: During the rest of the year, we still had a huge influence on the youth of Nenana. Russ and our youth pastor,

Kelvin Schubert, began Friday Youth Group. We were a couple of blocks away from the Living Center, where students from remote villages lived while attending our excellent high school. Far from home, most of the students had never experienced anything outside their tiny communities, and that included trains. They would run outdoors to see that amazing phenomenon when it roared through! Few had even seen passenger cars, most had only seen snow machines, or 4-wheelers as they were usually called, and pickup trucks. Some came from the windswept Arctic tundra, or the Aleutian Islands, where the biggest vegetation might be some willow brush. As I walked one young lady back to the Living Center after dark, she exclaimed how beautiful and tall our trees were! In the Interior of Alaska trees seldom grow very big, due to the long subzero winters. Some Black Spruce in permafrost areas are only a spindly 5 feet high after a hundred years. So, being the fountain of trivia that I am, I began to tell her about the redwoods of California, the REALLY big trees. I don't think she believed me…

Russ devised some crazy and amazing games that enthralled the young people, bonding them to new friends, and opening their hearts to the Gospel. Fortunately our rented home, which was also the church, had typical Alaskan varnished plywood floors, easily cleaned after a madhouse of bare feet plunged into pots of cold cooked spaghetti, mounds of shaving cream, and burst balloons. He encouraged teamwork between the youth of the Living Center and our own Nenana residents, and also challenged them. One of the favorite games was "Dunking for Dollars." Russ wadded up several one-dollar bills, a couple of fives, and sometimes a ten; put them in the bottom of a galvanized washtub; then filled it with bags of ice cubes and water. The object was to dunk your head into the icy mix, no hands allowed, and come up with prize money in your teeth.

OW!!! It was COLD! Even the Inuit (Eskimo) students came up screaming in chilly delight...

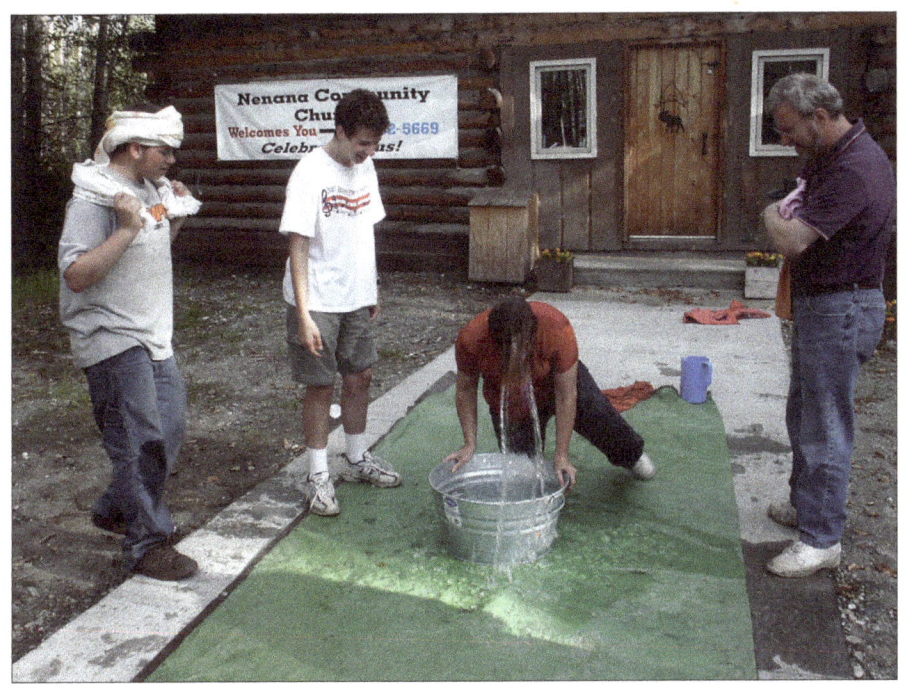

Dunking for Dollars

My youth pastor, Kelvin Schubert, came up with a mock quiz show of Bible knowledge, complete with buzzers. Some youth had never even seen a Bible before, much less opened and read one. Soon they were winning quizzes and asking questions about the stories. One I remember was a question about the twins born to Isaac and Rebekah: One loud answer was "Hairy Dude [Esau] and Mama's Boy [Jacob]!" Very original and very Alaskan, but very true! And best of all, many made professions of faith in Jesus Christ as their Lord.

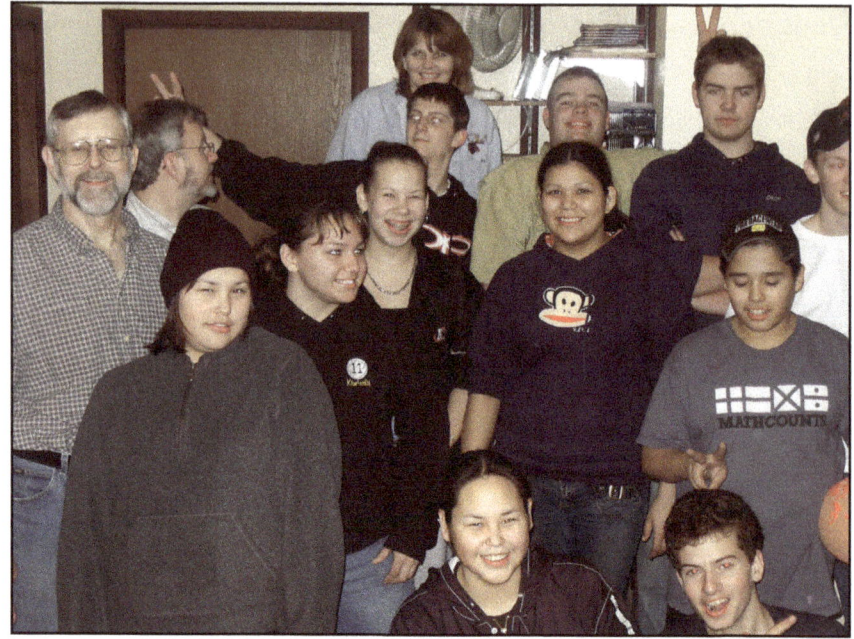

Youth Group with Russ, Kelvin Schubert and Vickie Turner

 Kelvin, his wife Ruth, and some of their children ran the AWANA Program, which we held in the Senior Center for the needed space. Village children flocked to it after school, just like the older students from the Living Center came to the youth group; many of their parents never went to church anywhere. But, as the children memorized Scripture to gain their badges, the parents had to help during the week, and heard the Gospel by osmosis. The influence of Nenana Community Church was spreading.

 Another thing Alice and I were adamant about, was getting involved in the daily life of our village. Flo Gierke's experience of not being able to contact a pastor in town when she needed one burned deep in our minds. We were determined everyone in the village would have reasonable access to godly counsel and prayer, so we opened our home as a public meeting place. Native ladies came for prayer on Wednesday evenings, youth group was Friday, and worship services were on Sunday. People would come and go at all hours. Alice and I substitute taught at the local high school, and I joined as a director on the library board, a vibrant little group run by Darcia Grace, which made sure all children had access to interesting books and year-round programs to help them develop an interest in reading. We participated in the Native Potlatches and got to know many of the elders and leaders of the village, and those who needed help. Because of our involvement with the elderly I was asked to join the board of directors of the Senior Center. One of my more interesting part-time jobs was being a jailer. We had two policemen in Nenana, one for day and one on night shift. Most of their time was spent patrolling Nenana and the segment of the George Parks Highway within the city limits. When there was someone in the jail cell, state law required that they be checked every 15 minutes and a log book kept up to date of all activities inside the jail. So, I was called in to help. I spent quite a few long nights listening to verbal abuse from an inebriated prisoner who wanted to get back to the local bars.

One of our first encounters was with a young Native man at a yard sale. He was looking at a hunting bow, and when we asked him what he would use it for he replied, "To shoot white men." When that didn't faze us, he entered into a conversation, although a bit inebriated. We offered him a ride home in our borrowed car. It was only a few blocks, but he didn't seem able to manage it on his own. So he picked up his 12-pack of Olympia beer, and sat in the passenger seat. After a block or two, he turned and looked at me suddenly, "Are you a cop?" No, I answered, not a cop. I guess some of my security persona still remained, but now I was interested in saving souls, not business assets.

After depositing him at his home, he invited us in and began a sentimental journey, showing us dusty photo albums of happier days. We saw pictures of his deceased mother whom he missed terribly, past seasons with his family at fish camp and hunting cabins, and his father who had recently died. You could see he was yearning for the outdoor life left behind many years ago. We had many further interactions with him; and are happy to say that he found the Lord, turned his life around, and is living with purpose today. We are still Facebook friends and happily comment on each other's lives.

Alice and I also made a point of having lunch at the Senior Center a few times a week, run by our "person of peace," Margaret Sanders. It was a favorite place for a delicious and inexpensive meal, often including local moose and salmon. Margaret introduced us to many leaders of the village, both Anglo and native, and taught us much of what we needed to know to function in the village. Then, in 2001 and much to my surprise, she began to introduce me to newcomers and tourists, who had discovered her lunches, as "Nenana's pastor." I knew then we were part of village life. God continued to work with her generous but no-nonsense spirit, and she soon made a profession of faith. Although she is gone now, her determination to serve the elders of the village will never be forgotten. When the inevitable summer forest fires filled the village with thick smoke, she would load up the Nenana Senior Center van with the village elders, and take them to air-conditioned motels in Fairbanks to protect their aging lungs. Many of the elderly owed their long lives to Margaret's selfless care at all hours.

It was at the Senior Center where we eventually met Bruce. Noticing a noisy clatter of dishes in the kitchen, and a new face at the pass-through window, we introduced ourselves to the blind man Margaret had employed as a helper. He was pleasant and capable, although we would sometimes nervously scan our sliced meats and salads for stray bits of finger. After our initial rental house was sold, in which we also held the Church, Margaret graciously offered us the use of the Senior Center on Sundays for our services, and for our weekday AWANA program. Bruce would listen to us attentively. Finally, one day he asked to speak with me. He wanted to know more about the Christ I was preaching, and then gave his life to the Lord. We did not have a baptismal, so I baptized him in the stock tank at the Assembly of God church on the edge of town. I then purchased the entire Bible on cassette tape and he listened to it daily. We often discussed it at his home after hours. He, too, has since gone to be with the Lord sometime after we left Alaska. And he is one of the precious souls that came into the Kingdom while we were there.

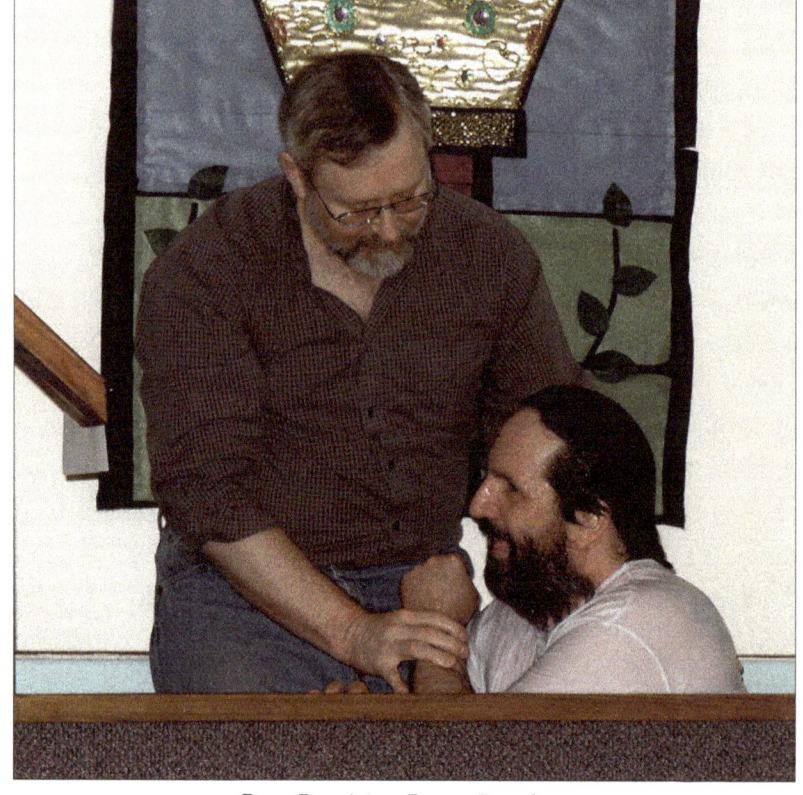

Russ Baptizing Bruce Boschert

Alice: Many of the village women found the long dark winters depressing, especially the Anglos whose husbands came there for jobs with the school or barge line. So, God led me to begin a ladies' ministry which I called "The Cabin Fever Club." We would meet once a month with a theme program, starting with a Bible devotional, then a craft or game and time of fellowship. Many of the women who normally never attended church would come to our aging log home, which WAS the church for years, and enjoyed that time together. The favorite month was February, when we had Chocolate Night, inspired by Valentine's Day. Once, Russ and I found inexpensive tickets to Geneva, Switzerland to visit my brother David. If you know anything about Swiss chocolate, and the "chocolatiers" found on almost every corner of the city, you will understand why we bought another small suitcase to bring home a big selection. Chocolate truffles, orange rind dipped in chocolate, and huge bars full of hazelnuts. Our trip was just before that year's Chocolate Night, and I think many will still remember it!

I also offered free painting and drawing lessons at the Cultural Center to the native youth, plus the village school (K-12); and the Living Center, where young people from remote villages came to board while attending our well-run high school. Many of the students had great talent which was going to waste without encouragement. I was happy to see one of my students take Junior Championship in Creative Arts at the Tanana Valley State Fair in Fairbanks. Another went on to Johns Hopkins University and is now a noted medical illustrator!

Chapter 7

Living the Wilderness Life

————†————

What was life like in a sleepy, little village in the interior of Alaska? Cold. In the winter at least. One morning Alice awakened me from sleep, telling me I needed to come outside with my camera. Our round outdoor thermometer had bottomed out at -60F. Other residents had experienced even colder weather in the past, below -70F. To put our winters into perspective, at -20F, the propane for our kitchen stove would not flow, so Alice cooked on the wood stove. At -50F, fuel oil for our furnace would gel, so back to the wood stove again. We usually cut and burned about 3-4 cords of firewood a year. Its heat really warmed us to the bone!

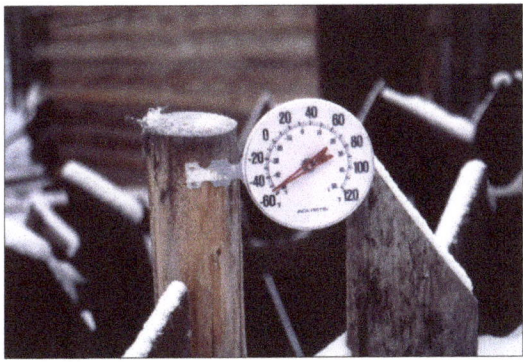

Winter is Cold!

We had to plug in our vehicle all night in subzero weather. There was a dipstick heater to keep the oil fluid; a battery blanket to keep it from freezing; and another heater on the transmission to keep that operational. And when it got to -50F, we were warned to not bother starting the engine, since the belts would snap from brittle cold. Getting into our car was another surprise for us as Cheechakos (newcomers). The foam seats were frozen as hard as rock; the tires were frozen flat on the bottom and took a few miles of thunk! thunk! thunk! to thaw and return to their original roundness. When we did go to Fairbanks, over an hour to the northeast, the supermarkets had electrical outlets at each parking space to keep their customers mobile. The city was in a low bowl surrounded by a ring of hills. Arriving before noon just as the sun rose, we often saw it blanketed in ice fog, glowing like a golden cloud. Our own village often had a cloud of ice fog overhead, which crystallized on every tree and twig like sparkling diamonds, and on the side of our log home too!

The interior is considered a cold desert. The snow rarely got much higher than mid-calf, and would not melt on sunny days, just evaporate, or sublimate, into the atmosphere. The powdery snow could be blown off our windshield in the morning, and the only real ice we usually saw was at the traffic light intersections in Fairbanks, where braking vehicles warmed it enough to form ice. Speaking of ice, I'll let Alice tell a story on herself.

Living the Wilderness Life

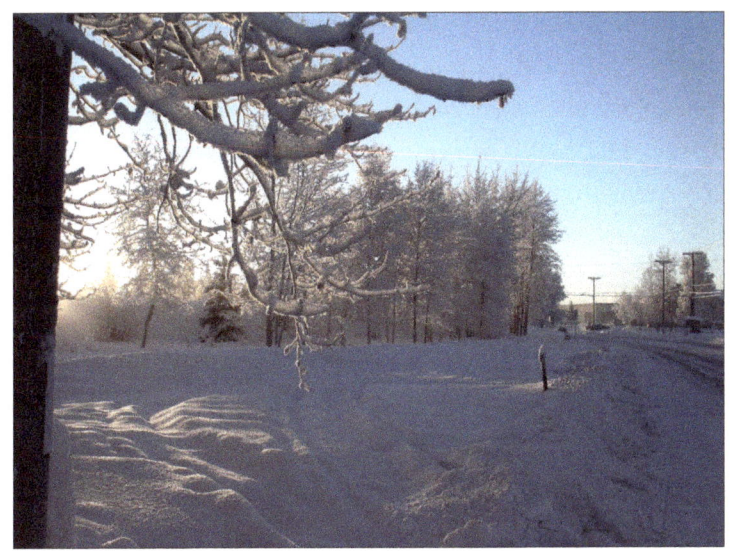

40 Below, Alaskan Interior

Alice: We were heading for Anchorage, six hours to the south, over the Alaska Range of mountains, to pick up our friend Vickie and her new husband Ed Pittman. They had been managing a store in the Aleutian Island chain and were coming back to the mainland for a while. By this time we had purchased a used 4WD crew cab GMC pickup; Russ was so happy that we could get out into wilder places with it for our outdoor adventures.

It must have been late January, since the sun was shining brightly and the Parks Highway was clear of any snow. Russ said he would take a nap while I drove the first lap and we headed south. The speed limit was 65, so of course I decided to set the cruise control on 67 so we would make good time. I went into autopilot mode, watching the spruce wilderness flash by. As we neared the village of Healy, just before the mountains, we topped a rise and a long stretch of black ice covered the pavement ahead. Yikes! I began to skid into oncoming traffic, then corrected to the right too sharply. In that area, the ground is marshy muskeg, so the road had been built up over fifteen feet high, maybe more. In a few seconds we were airborne over the side. The bump of the pavement edge awoke Russ a little, and I remember saying on the way down, "Oh, Russ, I am SO sorry I'm wrecking your truck!"

As always, the hand of God was with us. If we had gone down at right angles to the road, we would have nosedived into our radiator and probably flown through the windshield with fatal consequences. If we had gone down more parallel to the pavement, we would have rolled over on the steep bank with equally fatal consequences. As it was, we were on an approximately 45 degree angle, and the thick willow brush that grew on the bank slowed our descent. We somehow ended up facing north again, resting softly in the deep snow. Our German Shorthair Retriever in the back seat looked around in astonishment. Bumpy rides usually meant we were going on a hunting adventure in the back country, but this was a little much. I looked at Russ and he looked at me. "Are you OK?" we said in unison. No broken bones. No bruises. "Turn off the key!" he urged. I sheepishly admitted it was my fault, so I would climb up to the road and get a ride to call a wrecker. Cars had begun to pull over to check on us, and one offered to take me to nearby Healy and the gas station. On our way, I thanked God for not hitting the oncoming cars head-on, and they said. "We're glad too, because that was us! We saw you go over the edge and came back to see if you were OK."

Parks Highway Towing sent one of their expert men from Nenana, and 2 hours later, our snowy truck was up on the roadway again. Russ and the tow operator looked it over. Nothing appeared broken, no strange odors of brake fluid or anything else. He started it up, and it ran fine. I was so relieved,

"Let's go back home!" "Oh, no!" said Russ. "We're going to Anchorage. Vickie is expecting us, so it's time to get back in the saddle," and off we went. I will say I never used cruise control in the winter again.

Alaska was an outdoorsman's dream come true. But did we get to hunt and fish as often as we wanted? No. Ministry took most of our time, filling our days and often long hours into the night. But we did get to live on wonderful local moose meat (Alaskan beef) and delicious, fresh salmon. Alaskan moose are huge ungulates (a hoofed typically herbivorous quadruped mammal such as a pig, cow, deer, or horse); hitting one doesn't just dent your vehicle, it usually totals it and kills you. Their shoulders are level with a small car's roof, and the body mass is about the same as a Clydesdale horse, only on longer legs. It is an immovable object, when hit by a car or pickup truck.

Nenana is located on one of the few paved roads in this huge state, the George Parks Highway, and 18-wheel trucks ran up and down it between Anchorage and the North Slope oil fields. Unlike private cars, the tractor trailers won any confrontation with moose.

Alice: One semi we saw had "Here Moosie, Moosie!" written on its bug shield.

When a dead moose was reported, the State Police were anxious to have the huge carcass removed from the road as fast as possible to avoid further risks. Plus the state was very aware of the need to avoid waste; even if hit squarely on the hindquarters there was still potentially over 800 lbs. of delicious and nutritious meat, free of growth hormones and antibiotics. So, they have a "Roadkill List" usually made up of churches and community organizations. They go down the list in sequence calling phone numbers until someone answers "Yes, we'll get there ASAP."

We often got moose to clean and butcher especially in subzero weather when fingers freeze, carcasses stiffen, and few want to go out in the darkness. Our Youth Pastor Kelvin Schubert and I would go and retrieve the moose, then Alice and the two of us would have a two-day job ahead of us boning, grinding into burger, packaging, and freezing the meat.

Alice: We would field-dress the moose along the roadside, leaving that portion for the wolves and ravens to clean up. Then we'd load it on Kelvin's little trailer with much grunting and pushing. If it were not subzero weather, we would hang it from a tree in our yard, skin it, and then move the carcass into our church/home onto a large sheet of heavy plastic. Indoors was better in winter due to numbing cold; and in summer due to tormenting swarms of mosquitos and flies. I would start cutting it up, boning the meat, and putting major chunks into the fridge. Kelvin would grind all the smaller pieces, and Russ would wrap and freeze everything.

We wasted nothing, Tongue, liver, heart, kidneys, and brains. Then came the sharing. Russ and I and Kelvin's family had some, but we always gave a quarter of the moose either to the Senior Center or to the Native Corporation to feed needy elders. Older Native women wanted the legs and feet for soup; and the head went to the Native community for the first course of every Potlatch, Moose Nose Soup. The huge pile of leftover bones went to our neighbors, Gopher and Karen Lord, who cooked them up with their homemade sled dog feed. The skins went to a young Native man who was documenting and following the Old Ways. Alex Ketzler would brain tan and smoke the hides, then make useful items. I have a pair of beaded moccasins he crafted and edged with dark beaver fur. A work of art, and still fragrant from the aspen smoking process.

But we did hunt, fish and enjoy the spectacular wilderness around us! Denali (Mt. McKinley) is the highest mountain in North America looming high above the Alaska Range 120 miles to our south. Since it is so much taller than anything around it, it has its own weather system, often covered by a bank of thick clouds. It is only visible about 30% of the year. When it is, village people spread the news, "The Mountain is out!"

So I began to think of Denali as an allegory of God. We hear the stories that a Great Being exists, but we cannot see Him. After a time we begin to doubt, since all we see is the bank of dim clouds rising above all the 10,000+ ft. snowy peaks. Then one clear day, suddenly, unexpectedly, there it is!

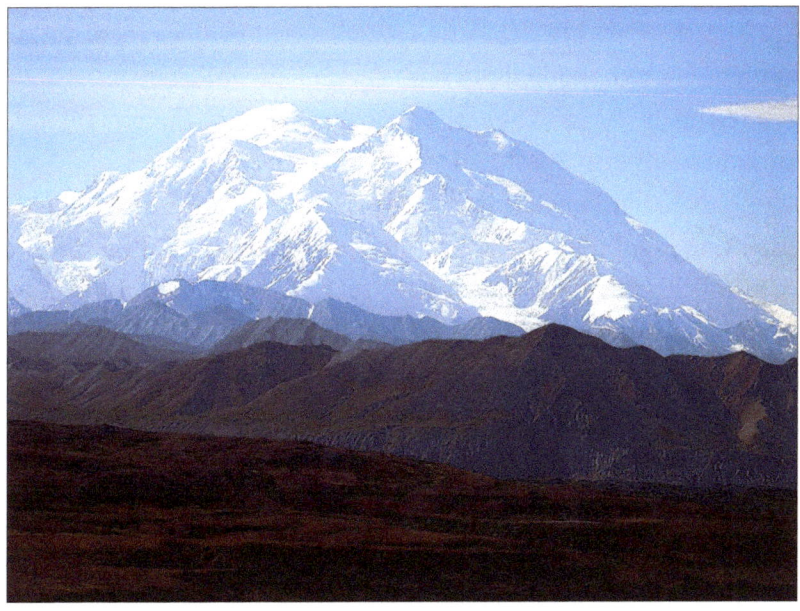

Denali, The Great One

Ascending majestically above all else, in rock solid reality on the southern horizon, the Great One at 20,230 feet of breathtaking, snow covered beauty. So it is with the Lord. We see nothing happening and begin to doubt our prayers are even being heard. Then He acts! And His majesty is unmistakable as He impacts our lives.

Movies show rushing rivers cascading over rocks in their Alaskan adventures, usually filmed in Alberta or Oregon. In reality, Alaska's major rivers formed a huge inland waterway system, the Yukon, Tanana, Koyukuk, Kantishna and Kuskokwim. They are glacier fed, the color of milky tea, and deceptively flat and slow looking. When we watched logs rushing downstream, we realized the swiftness of the current. Treacherous bars of glacial silt and huge piles of dead spruce further complicated river travel. Some of the trees, broken free during the crashing of ice floes in spring breakup, stuck to the bottom on one end, and the free end bobbing just beneath the surface threatening death to unwary boaters. The local radio station, KIAM, made daily reports on river water levels, which tended to flood in August, when the glaciers melted fastest. Freight to all the remote villages built along the rivers came by barge. Nenana boasted two barge lines, the larger Yutana, and the more local one owned by Mr. and Mrs. Jahola. Fuel oil for heating, gasoline for generators, pickups and snow machines, dog food for the racing teams, flour, milk, bread and toilet paper all had to be delivered before freeze-up. Despite having no roads leading to them, many remote villagers had pickup trucks, used on the 5 or six miles of local dirt roads into the forest.

When winter came and the river ice was four feet thick, the rivers were used for highways. Riding on the Tanana River ice was faster going up to Fairbanks by snow machine than taking the winding Parks Highway over the Tanana Hills. The

Arctic village of Bettles had truck freight in the winter. It was in the marshy tundra, with no road connection in summer. But in winter, they made an "ice bridge" over the Koyukuk River, pumping upriver water onto the ice to thicken it so tractor trailers could cross safely. Then they rolled over the hard frozen tundra to and from Fairbanks. Winter travel was often more efficient than summertime.

On one moose hunting trip we took up the Kantishna River with Percy Duyck, a veteran river man, he carefully made his way between and over silt bars, his eyes glued on the river surface for telltale signs of logs and other hazards; then let us off at the mouth of Lynx Creek so we could canoe up to the wilderness cabin we rented from Ruth and Larry Coy. His boat was a beautiful testimony to his cabinet making skills, but could go no further since the water levels were unusually low that year. We carried our gear and drinking water cans up the steep cliff and finally, wearily, left some of it under a tarp at the Creek's edge. Our friends from Maryland, Dan and Cindy Ellis, shared the experience with us. Although we never saw a moose, the trip was a true wilderness adventure, 200 miles from the nearest road. We slept in the well-built cabin crafted from huge white spruce logs. Alice cooked and Cindy cleaned up, while Danny and I scouted for elusive moose, but only saw pink grizzly bear scat filled with autumn cranberries. As eagles flew above us, Cindy shot grouse which Alice cooked for dinner on our portable camp stove. Our friends saw their first Northern Lights on the long walk to the outhouse, which was outfitted with a thick blue foam seat, so our bottoms would not freeze to the wood. Then to cap it off, after a night of hard frost, we began to hear a strange sound in the distance. Soon, thousands upon thousands of Sandhill cranes, in wave after wave, passed overhead on their southward migration. That experience alone was worth the trip.

This trip taught us the magnitude of the Alaskan wilderness. Far from any trace of civilization, except what we had carried in a small boat, we began to realize how insignificant mankind is in the scheme of things. In an urban environment, among busy crowds of our own kind, it is easy to believe we are important to the events of earth. Out in the middle of the Great Land, its mountains and forests and rivers, God's Creation speaks silently but forcefully that He is the center of the universe, and we are but tiny mortals, dots in the landscape. Very humbling.

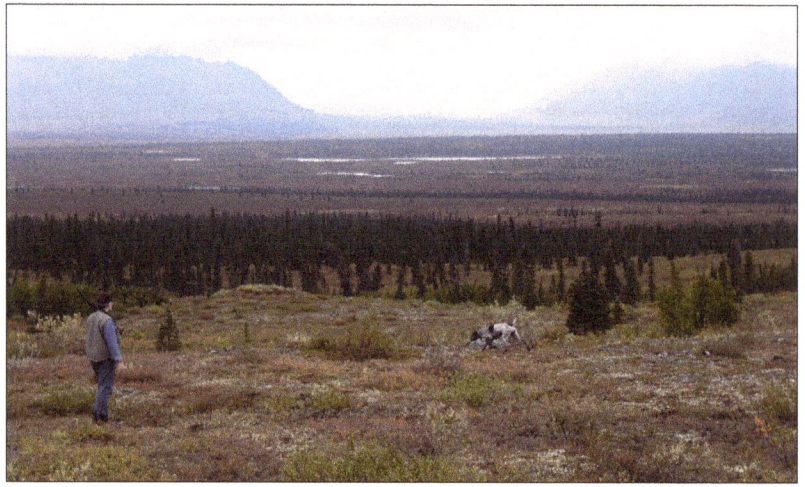

Russ Hunting on the Alaskan Tundra

Alice and I hunted ruffed grouse each autumn as the aspens turned to gold among the dark spruce. And each August, we went south to Wasilla and the Little Susitna River for 2 or 3 thrilling days of Silver Salmon fishing, filling our freezer for the winter with huge fish fresh from the ocean. By the time salmon came up to Nenana, they had travelled over 1000 miles up the Yukon and Tanana river system. Our neighbors caught hundreds of them in huge fish wheels, but we preferred the excitement of hook and line. No fruit trees grew north of the Alaska Range, but the Lord provided many square miles of wild berries, strawberries, raspberries, highbush cranberries, lowbush cranberries frequented by grouse, and incredibly delicious blueberries. The alpine tundra blueberries are not round, but grapelike; a bit tart but with the most intense blueberry flavor. But since they are also loved by black and grizzly bears, I insisted that Alice wear a .44 magnum revolver as part of her gear when going out with the Native ladies to pick berries.

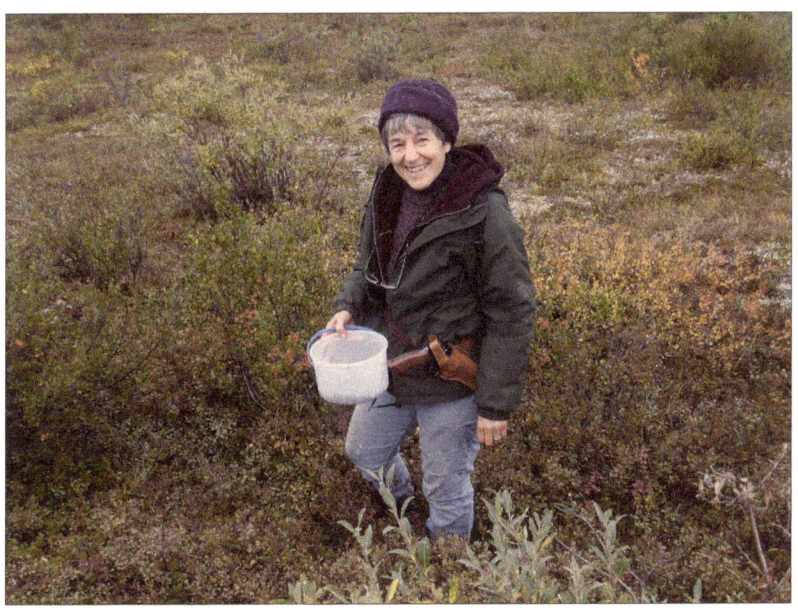

Alice Berry-picking, with Bear Insurance

Alice: Life was good. Russ and I shared moose, salmon, black bear, grizzly bear, caribou, wild sheep, and even an unfortunate porcupine with our friends, and the more adventurous of summer Mission Team members. Summers were cool and filled with long days of sunlight. We could not see stars from

April through late August. Wildflowers burst out everywhere, racing to produce seed in the short growing season. Wild roses filled roadsides and forest edges; succeeded by marshes filled with blue iris. And when the pink fireweed bloomed to the top of its stem, we knew frost was near. By then the nights were dark again and the Northern lights danced across the stars. Despite the millions of mosquitos, we were in an earthly version of Paradise. This was the adventure I meant in my personal advertisement so long ago, and I was sharing it with the love of my life.

Our current pastor, John Dickey, likes to remind us that "The Accuser is working against us day and night." And sure enough, even though it seemed everything was going well, trouble struck a mighty blow. In 2002, I was diagnosed with laryngeal cancer. The doctor performed surgery and applied radiation therapy for five and one-half weeks. Following the radiation treatment, I could not talk or preach for the next several months.

Soon after, my father fell ill and passed away. I flew to Maryland, unable to do more than whisper. Two weeks after the death of my father, my mother passed away. We were returning from my Dad's funeral at Arlington National Cemetery when I received a phone call that I had better come right away. My mother would not last through the night. And finally, in the fall of that same year, my grandmother quietly went home to be with the Lord at the young age of 101. It was the prayers and love of both my parents and grandmother that caused me to turn my life around with a new desire to seek the Lord. I do miss them terribly! And I am so grateful that God allowed them to live long enough to see me actively serving Him.

Alice: Early in that year, we had discussed asking for a summer missionary to help us with the mushrooming AWANA and Youth Group ministries of our church, and the Basketball Camp just prior to the beginning of the new school year. The two replies presented a dilemma; both were excellent candidates. Which one should we choose? I finally suggested to Russ that we accept both of them. He questioned whether we would have enough work to keep two summer missionaries busy, but finally assented. Little did we know how much we would need them both! Doug Ledbetter, Oklahoma Baptist University student, and son of friends at Midwestern Baptist Seminary, became a dynamic youth leader. Vickie Turner, recommended by Pastor William Gunter and his wife Becky, was a tremendous help to me during Russ' absence for his parents' funerals. She was as capable with a chain saw as with children's ministry. While I was busy getting pulpit supply for the church on Sundays, she helped me survive all the work and worry. The ministry of Nenana Community Church was written up in the Southern Baptist Convention's national news publication, the Baptist Press, twice! An article about our ministry was even published in a denominational newspaper in the Netherlands a few months later. By the way, in 2003 Vickie returned to Alaska as a house parent at the Living Center; and on one of her school-sponsored trips to Nome to visit with parents of our students, she met the man who is now her husband!

Sickness, loss, and hardship; that whole year was harsh and difficult. But as God had promised, if we trust in Him with our whole heart, He would straighten the path before us. And so, we kept going. Now, "straight paths" sometimes take unexpected twist and turns, even though they result in reaching God's goals.

Chapter 8

The Call of South Asia

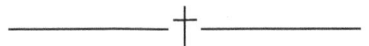

One day, while we were still in Alaska, I received an email from Pastor Johnpaul of Tenali, India. He stumbled upon the small website I had put on the internet to keep supporters informed of the progress of our work. And in 2001, he sent me an email. All that he wrote was his name and a short introduction to his ministry. And then he asked, "Would you please come to India and preach to my people?"

Alice was skeptical. Surely this was one of those "Nigerian" email schemes trying to swindle us out of some money. I was not so sure, and so I started an email dialogue with him. Alice and I prayed and talked. And we talked and prayed. Finally, after two years we decided to take the chance, and in 2003 we boarded a plane for our first short-term mission trip to the subcontinent of India. It was an incredible experience! We fell in love with the country, and God put a love in our hearts for the people. And from that time forward we traveled to India over the next ten years, ministering in villages, training pastors, teaching children, and encouraging the local church.

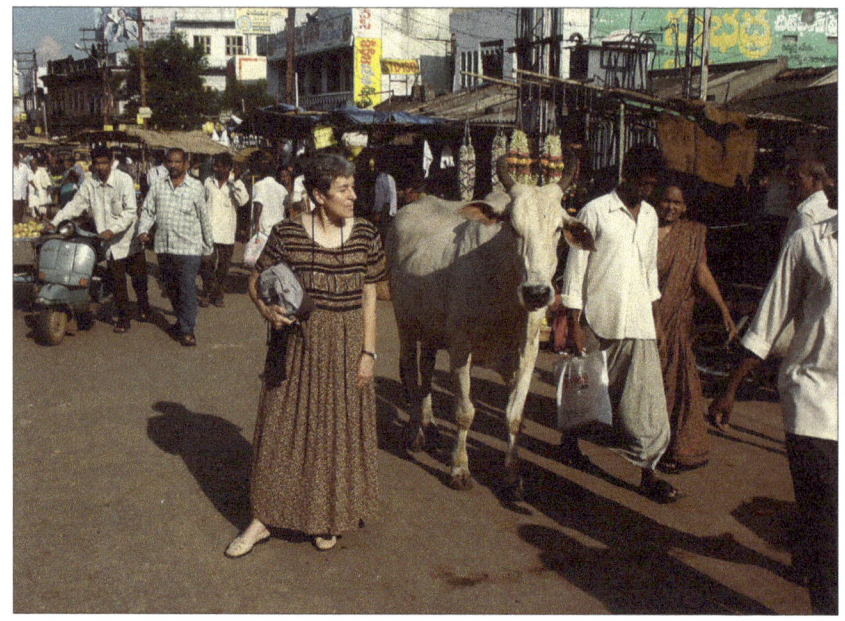

Alice Experiencing A New Culture

Alice: Yes, I was very skeptical. And reluctant to go to the Third World. People in Fairbanks considered Nenana a "Third World Country" and often wondered aloud why we ever moved there; but it was our dream come true, life at the edge of pristine wilderness. The true Third World I had heard about was a place of filth, disease, suffering, poverty and innumerable people, not the spruce-scented air, pure water and uncrowded, boreal forests of Alaska. I knew I would see terrible things I could not "fix" and I cringed from subjecting my emotions to them. But Russ and God finally convinced me to go. The conditions were often terrible but we grew to love the people, the Lord loved them, created them, and wanted them in His Kingdom. His goal is His glory among all the nations, and we are sent to fulfill that goal.

I remember looking down on the city of Hyderabad as we came in for our first landing. It had 6 million people, but the old airport was about the size of the small one in Fairbanks. And it smelled heavily of mildew and non-functional toilets. My heart sank further as we emerged into the night with our host. More "unique aromas" assailed me, especially that of sun ripened human urine. We were taken to the "Tulip Deluxe Hotel" near the Shamshabad Train Station, squeaked up to our floor in a creaky freight style elevator, and shown to a room. Jet lag wouldn't let me sleep, so I spent time observing our surroundings. The thin mattress had some ragged sheets on it, and the western toilet in the bathroom had a shower head on a cable instead of toilet paper; it dripped constantly. At least it was better than the standard Indian toilet, which is a bowl set at floor level, requiring squatting and careful balancing. We were warned never to drink from the carafe of water on the rickety night table. I looked out the window and saw big black garbage bags below, obviously trash put out for pickup. When they rolled over I saw that these were the street poor, and the garbage bags their only shelter, even in the heavy monsoon rains. As morning approached, I heard the cacophony of Indian traffic, chaos at its finest, growing louder. Men urinated against walls as women in flowing saris hurried to their destinations among the swarms of buses, taxis, auto rickshaws and bicycles—all honking their horns and bells. Ragged beggars sat at the gates of countless temples and shrines of idolatry. I was definitely in another world.

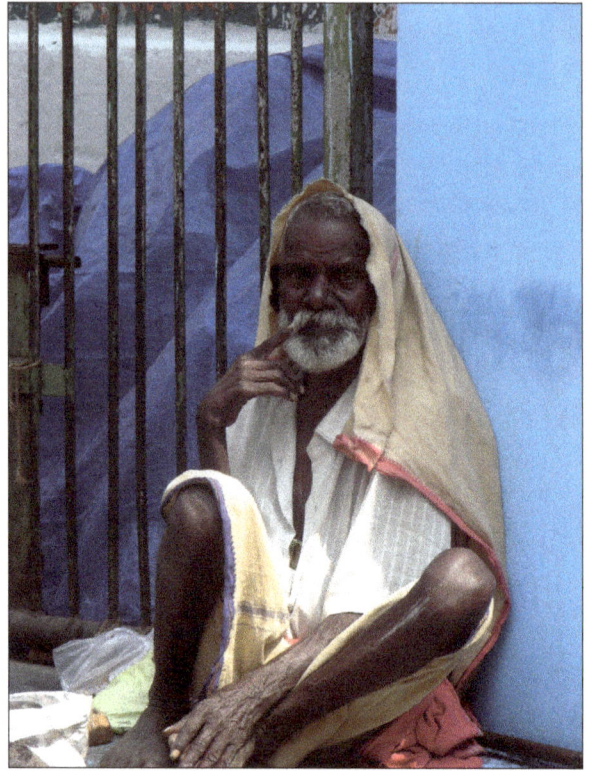

Beggar at a Temple Gate

From that day on, we began the process of adapting ourselves to many a church in tiny thatch huts and breathlessly hot air when the inadequate power grid—and thus the ceiling fans—of India failed almost daily. Russ was so much taller than most of the rural people, that he banged his head against the structural poles when he stood up to preach. The church members sat cross-legged on the floor on woven mats with women and children on the preacher's right, men on the left. The walls were also woven palm mats, sometimes plastered with a mixture of cow dung and mud. Tithes were a precious cupful of rice poured into a large bowl beneath the altar, for the pastor and his family to live on for the week.

People lined up for prayer afterward; with goiter, malarial fevers, sick children, and so many other maladies that were easily treatable in the United States. Some fell at Russ' feet in worship, but he hastily lifted them up, saying, "Not me, but the Lord I serve!" Sometimes we ran out of time in the night, so I ended up with an armful of ladies for a group prayer. We went after dark to avoid confrontation with the Hindu authorities who did not condone preaching Christ to their people. Recently, under the current anti-Christian Prime Minister, many states have passed anti-conversion laws. Once born a Hindu, always a Hindu. Once born into a caste, whether rich and high, or low and miserable, that is where you stay, forever. In their minds the only way out was "reincarnation."

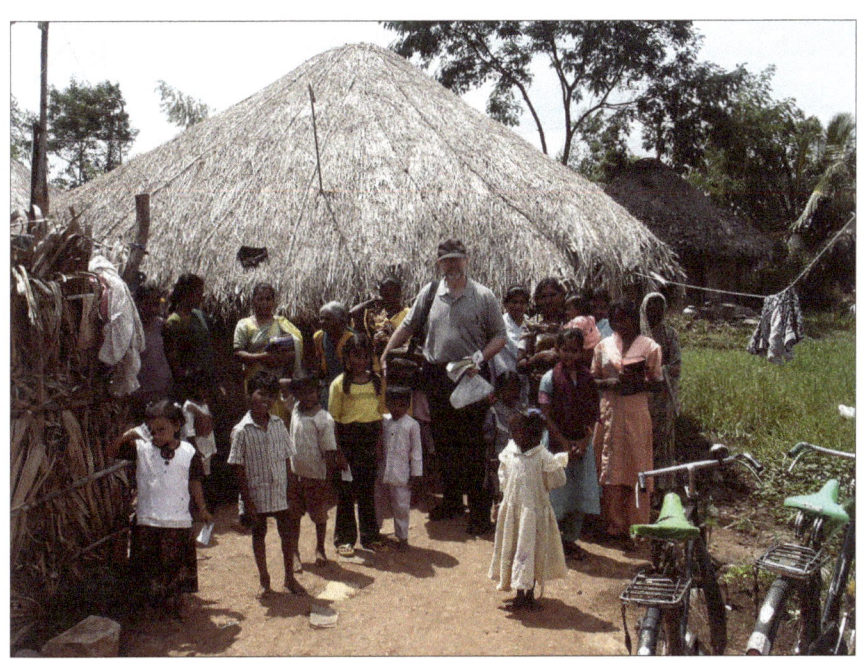

Russ after service, Thatch Church

We gave out blankets to widows, outcast, pitiful, and abandoned souls with no property rights, who lived on the streets or slept in friendly churches, and Bibles, more precious than food or blankets. We ministered to lepers and HIV/AIDS victims. I personally never quite got used to the huge amounts of chili peppers used in south India cooking. No matter how I begged, and even bought veggies in the street markets, and asked for plain boiled food, they never could serve it without lots of chili. Mine was merely a three-alarm fire instead of a five-alarm!

When we returned to Nenana from those trips, the silk saris I brought back dazzled their eyes. I sold them at fundraisers and used the money to support our ministry to India. This went on for the next ten years.

Eventually the time came when God told us to move on. Nenana Community Church was left with a building lot next to the school, since much of our ministry centered on children and youth, and a solid foundational structure for the future. The church is still going strong today under the capable leadership of Pastor William Troxel and his lovely wife, Rebecca.

Upon leaving Alaska, we relocated to Clifton Forge, Virginia. We spent four months living there and attending Clifton Forge Baptist Church, where we began an evangelism and outreach program.

Alice: We had been on our way to join an international campus ministry in Blacksburg VA. Although we loved Bob and Sandra Jackson, from our Galax days, we were having second thoughts about our specific role there. As we neared the West Virginia/Virginia line, our dashboard began to smoke. It was dusk, and our headlight switch was burning up. We could find nowhere to park our pickup and U-Haul trailer, so we limped into Covington VA and a cheap motel. At a restaurant that evening, the people at the next table raved about the area, and we began to think we didn't really HAVE to go onward. Let's admit to our friends that we don't believe we are a good fit for children's ministry; just stay here and see what God has ahead of us. So we went into Clifton Forge and looked for a place to rent temporarily while we rested and regrouped after the long road trip from Alaska.

Even though we were only there a short while, we made lasting friendships in those Allegheny Mountains. We picked wild blueberries, hiked along the mountain creeks, and spent time with Kae and Larry Lacy in their cabin along the Cowpasture River, which joined the Jackson River to form the beloved James River of Virginia's history and ours.

We had been praying concerning God's will for our life and ministry when we received a call to Idaho to revitalize two dying churches that were hurting, and desperate for healing. At the First Baptist Church, Gooding, ID I began to think God had brought me there only to bury people. Within the first 6-8 months I officiated eight funerals, and they weren't even all members. After reorganization, producing a "Policies & Procedures Manual," starting regular Wednesday night Bible study and prayer time, and doing evangelism training the church began to turn around and grow. Both churches are still going strong today.

Alice: I think that our most enjoyable ministry there was with the Youth Groups Russ started. I remember our second date, when we promised each other that we would never grow up, and I think that aspect carried over into our success with youth wherever we ministered. Russ invited singing groups and an amazing Christian ventriloquist. We held harvest parties in the parking lot for the entire community. We also had a vibrant ministry with the many Hispanics who worked in the irrigated farmlands and huge dairies and cheese factories of Idaho. I often walked with ladies from the rundown trailer park across from the church, learning more Spanish every day. We began a Hispanic Bible Study in our double-wide parsonage, since they were reluctant to enter a Protestant church. At first, we had two Spanish-speaking helpers. Later I led it myself with God's grace. Many lives were changed and we still have friends from those days. Imagine sitting in an old rented mobile home, reading a Spanish Bible about the story of Ruth, with a lady called Naomi who was just discovering who she had been named after! Sweet memories!

We fell in love with Idaho. The sagebrush desert, seemingly barren, was filled with life of its own. I remember being out with Russ, just after sunset, running our GSP Gypsy several miles north of Rupert. The sky was still rose-grey with last light in the west, a huge evening star glowing near the horizon, distant coyotes taking up their serenade. Pungent sage aroma filled the deepening night as the moon rose silver on a dry and lonely land.

And then there were the mountains! After a long week of ministry and visitation and counseling, youth group on Fridays, and church on Sundays, we would take Mondays as our day off. With our little travel trailer behind the Jeep, we'd look for a wild place to spend the next 24 hours. Sometimes it was on the side of a creek in the Bennet Hills overlooking the Camas Prairie below. We loved those wetlands, especially in early spring when migratory waterfowl flocked in amazing numbers and variety on their way north. There stilts, avocets, ibis, curlew, willet, snipe and so many more—including resident

Sandhill crane returning to their nesting grounds. And then around Memorial Day, the entire area was covered with purple Camas blossoms, an amazing display of God's Creation!

A little further up the dirt road, we found a spring seep thick with miner's lettuce, an oasis among the rock formations of a high and dry country. Russ had his camera out, and suddenly called me over. A praying mantis had captured a tiny lizard! He has photos to prove it.

Another favorite place was Pioneer Creek, on Federal land north of Sun Valley. Camping was free at any place with an established fire ring, an amazing way to enjoy God's country just beyond the multimillion dollar vacation homes of the rich and famous. We would pull off along the rushing mountain stream, surrounded by the fir forest, and enjoy the peaks of the Sawtooth Mountains high above us. What peace and solitude! It was the perfect place to restore our souls for another week of dealing with the church flock, the community, and all its pain and problems.

Russ and I hiked the canyons, tent-camped in the desert, hunted and ate jackrabbit, saw elk and antelope on the ridges and in the volcanic rock formations. All that time his legs and feet pained him terribly, and he had to rest often before going on. The doctors had said it was peripheral neuropathy and nothing could be done. If only we had known.

We tried to stay in Idaho after our ministry was over, but it was too expensive. The mountains had lured moneyed celebrities from Hollywood and elsewhere, and we just could not afford the resulting prices. Then, exhausted from all the hard work, we began to prayerfully research possible communities to put down roots.

Chapter 9

Retirement—Or Is It?

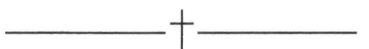

During our extensive research into a suitable place to retire, Oklahoma came to the forefront due to low cost of living, and I began to look for a job of some type to give us a chance to get settled in. I found a listing online for a managerial position with a storage rental facility in the university town of Stillwater. It didn't pay a great deal but a small apartment was part of the pay package.

One of the things I learned a long time ago was that God has a sense of humor. Making my way to the interview, following detailed directions to the facility, I ran into some road construction that forced me to detour and pass right by the only Southern Baptist church I saw on that side of town. After the interview I was informed I had the job but I had to be there in two weeks or less. Wow, this was unexpected! We hadn't even started packing yet. In fact, I hadn't even mentioned to the church I was leaving! On the way to the airport I called Alice to let her know I got the job and we needed to start packing, immediately! She picked me up upon my arrival in Boise on Saturday and four days later we were on the road to

Oklahoma, where we were hoping to retire. As usual, we soon realized that God had other plans for our future.

After we got settled into my new job and the apartment, it was time to look for a new church home. I had seen Hillcrest Baptist Church on the detour to my initial interview. So it seemed like a good place to start. We would check out other churches on following Sundays. Our first Sunday there was awesome! We have visited many different churches around the U.S. and a few in other countries. But this one was authentically friendly. The people welcomed us with open arms and twelve years later we are still members here; we never checked out any others. God had led us "by accident" to Hillcrest Baptist—a church with a missionary heart. Here, we healed from the wounds of spiritual battle and turned our thoughts back to India. It was reborn as the central focus in our life.

Respected friends suggested we consider starting a charitable organization to broaden our donor base and enlist other people in what had been a personal ministry for many years. As we began praying through this idea and talking to some of our long-time supporters, we began to see God's hand moving. Many people told us it would take over six months for the paperwork to be approved by the Internal Revenue Service. Yet, we received our approval within three months. As we talked to people about the new mission organization I could sense the growing excitement in what God was doing, and the funds began to flow in. One of the first items of business was to convince at least three people of the value of serving as Board of Directors. Of course, we couldn't pay anyone, but God would surely bless them for their compassion and generous spirit. My hope was that I would find men and women of good character, strong in their faith, and willing to tell me when I was going in the wrong direction with the organization. Within a short time I had not only the three required directors, but six additional volunteers. The exact number I had prayed that God would provide. So, in early 2008, Asia International Mission was born and we returned to the place we had seen God leading us and working in a dark and hurting land. One would think that after twelve years of God blessing our ministry I would expect nothing less than a continual working of the Holy Spirit in all we were doing. Yet, as usual, I remained amazed as God opened door after door into the individual lives and communities of the people of India, and a continual reminder that if only we would "Trust in the LORD with all your heart...he will make your paths straight." (Proverbs 3:5-6) A children's home was built on the south side of Tenali in the state of Andhra Pradesh. Churches were planted in unreached villages throughout several other states. We distributed Bibles and gospel tracts, and wherever we traveled our hosts arranged village-wide meetings where the Good News was preached to people who had never heard the name of Jesus. We knew without a doubt we were where God wanted us to be.

Since the beginning of my ministry, my philosophy has been based on the three points of the triangle. At the top point is the spiritual (God), the bottom right point is the physical (food, shelter, clean water, etc.), and the bottom left point is mental (education of all types). So based on this philosophy we have worked to provide housing and medical care where we are financially able.

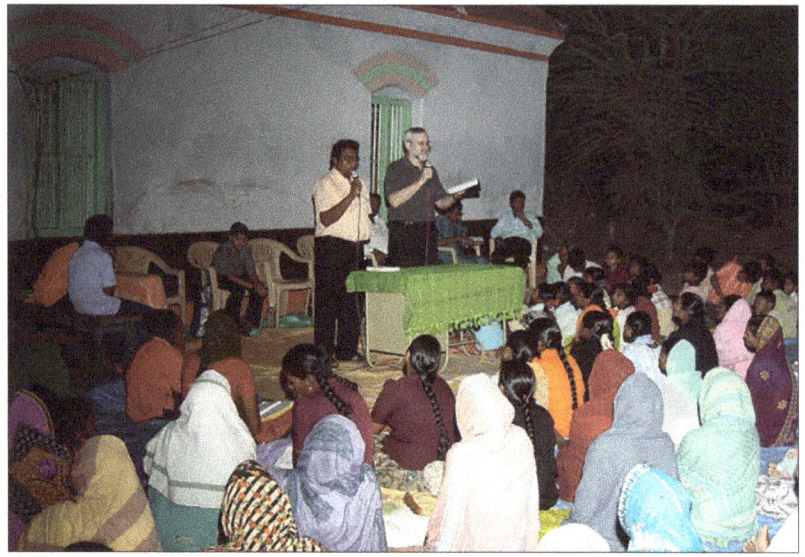

Russ preaching a village Gospel meeting

Another dire need in India, in fact worldwide, is pure water. Thousands of children die each day due to waterborne diseases and parasites, and adults are also affected by the millions. So, water wells became another physical help to the people where God led us.

During this time everything was going great! I was on top of the world. People were responding to the gospel, children were being given a chance at a better life, and God was good! Yet once again, trials and troubles struck! Our life verse says that "He will make your paths straight…" and that's true. Yet, the enemy continued to ambush and harass us at every step along that path, trying to stop us from carrying the gospel to those who are firmly entangled in his evil grasp.

Now, many believers think that once we begin following Christ everything will be wonderful. God will always be there to catch us; if we need healing, God will heal us, and He will provide for our every want and need. But you see, God never promised that we would be free from suffering in this life.

His promise was, "I have told you these things, so that in me you may have peace. In this world, you will have trouble. But take heart! I have overcome the world." (John 16:33) No matter the struggles we are dealing with, we can always be certain that God has won the battle, and will carry us through to the end.

Several years before, Alice and I had been hiking near Galax, VA on a trail that took us along the New River. This is a favorite hiking, boating, and fishing spot for both local people and adventurers. I began to have pain in my left foot and it eventually spread to my right foot. Over the next 18 years, several different doctors attempted to diagnose the problem. We prayed for healing and continued to consult with various doctors. Yet, there was no healing, and even though we consulted a variety of specialists in several different states, no one was ever able to diagnose the cause of the pain.

During the March 2009 mission trip back to India, as I was speaking one Sunday morning in Brother Isaac's church, I knelt down to illustrate God forming man from the dust and breathing life into him. When I stood, a sharp, stabbing pain gripped my right leg, and I fell to the floor! Six of the men carried me downstairs. They took me to a local doctor for diagnosis, and as we entered the door to his office, I noticed a book on his desk that said "1001 Home Remedies" by Reader's Digest, and I thought, "Is this where I really want to be?"

The doctor examined me and determined that in his best judgment I had a blood clot. So, he gave me some super aspirin and sent me back to Brother Johnpaul's house. In the meantime, Alice had contacted our family physician back in the U.S., who was originally from India. The doctor told her that I needed to immediately go to a "real" hospital in Hyderabad, about a six-hour train ride north of Tenali. So, after wrapping up most of my ministry obligations in Tenali, I headed north by train.

Alice: What Russ neglected to mention was that Dr. Sharma said this was a "life-threatening" event and to get to a major city hospital, ASAP! "Wrapping up" means he worked for 3 more days, then took the long train ride. MEN! Can't get them to a doctor except on a stretcher.

After arriving in Hyderabad, the capital of Andhra Pradesh, I found myself at the Wockhardt Kamenini Heart Hospital. It was one of the better-known hospitals in India specializing in Cardiology. A Doppler scan revealed strings of many aneurysms, which are swellings and constrictions, in the arteries behind both knees. They had been forming clots for over 15 years; filling my leg and foot arteries with tiny, but deadly, little blood clots, starving my feet of oxygen and causing irreparable damage to them. Dr. Chandrashekar attempted bypass surgery, but it was unsuccessful due to the extensive damage already caused by the blood clots. So, they sewed me up, told me to go home, take blood thinners and hope for the best.

Alice: This was the one time I had not accompanied Russ to India; I was headed for Honduras on a Mission Trip to a Spanish-speaking country at long last. We had done so much work with Hispanics in the US, but I had never been south of the border.

When Russ called about his blood clot and upcoming surgery, I was deeply concerned and I needed to be by his side. Hastily I purchased tickets to India, routed through Houston so I could pick up my visa at the Indian Consulate during a 12-hour layover. I had someone take me to the OKC airport and stood in line, only to be told I could not board the plane for an international destination unless I already had my visa. No pleading or argument would change their minds. So I went home in despair. My driver, Queena Dickey, asked if I had prayed about this trip. No, I replied, I just knew I had to be there! Not a good answer.

Somehow I obtained an in-country flight to Chicago, and then a separate international flight to India. I had enough time to go to the Indian Consulate there and purchase an emergency visa. When I arrived, I stepped out of the airport, and the taxi waiting right in front of me had an Indian driver! Was this not God's doing? The driver knew exactly where the independent agency was for visa applications, drove me there, and waited patiently. First, they said I had to take my luggage and leave it down the street at a department store since they would not allow it in their

building. So I hurriedly ran down the street and checked my luggage, with only a few minutes of office time remaining. When I came back, they informed me that they could not give me a visa, since I lived in Oklahoma, and had to go through Houston. Besides, they were closing in a few minutes. Panic! I went out in the hallway and finally prayed fervently to the Lord. I came back to plead with them. By this time I was in tears. They melted at long last and let me apply for the visa. Then I was driven by the ever-patient taxi man to the Indian Consulate and received my document. The driver got me back to O'Hare in plenty of time for my flight to India. Needless to say, I tipped him handsomely. God had worked through him to get me to Russ.

When I arrived in Hyderabad, some of Russ' Indian friends came to pick me up. He was staying at the Tourist Palace, a local hotel which was a palace in name only, but adequate. He was giving himself prescribed heparin shots to prevent further clots during the upcoming surgery and his body was full of dark bruises. We checked into the hospital and I was allowed to stay in his room, a common practice in India where family is expected to care for the patient. The narrow bench at least had a vinyl cushion to sleep on. Indian physicians are very competent, even with aging equipment, but the cleanliness of the hospital left a little to be desired. The light fixture hung from the hole in the ceiling, where lizards darted in and out. The windows did not close properly, the screens were ragged, and the faded curtains sagged from their rods. The room was swabbed with disinfectant each day which made me happy. But the drain in the bathroom had moth balls piled in it to deter some of the swarms of gnats that hovered there.

When I went down to eat in the cafeteria, the servers noted that I was a foreigner since it was hard to hide the fact. So instead of the everyday stainless steel plates, they pulled a fancy china plate from under the counter, wiped it with a dusty leaf of old newspaper, and served me my meal in style; which I wish they hadn't. I will say that their fruit salad was the best I have ever eaten; Russ ordered it often. It was a medley of fresh grapes, figs, pineapple, mango and many other delectables. During the several pre-op days, we had a Muslim floor doctor. She spoke Urdu and English, and observed us carefully every day. Finally she spoke up and said she had heard that all American marriages were bad, but that we obviously had a good marriage. We told her it was because the Lord was the head of our marriage, which made her think. Russ and I prayed that she would be drawn to the Messiah. I had the opportunity to speak with another Muslim lady in the waiting area whose mother was close to death. She did not object to my praying with her in Jesus' Name, and I pray that she, too, would be influenced by her daughter's Christian school to find the Lord.

When the time came for Russ to go into surgery, we prayed together. And his Indian friends who spent much time in our room prayed as well, then mentioned that as a pastor, one of them expected to be given a little monetary gift for his prayer. Such is life in India.

Since the operation would take hours, I waited and paced, then went out for one of my usual walks on the grounds. The security guards at the entrance gate to the hospital had questioned me the first day, worried that I was an escaping patient who would not pay my bill. I had to explain that I needed the exercise, and my husband was a patient on the third floor. When I returned, our friends said Russ was already in recovery! What was happening? They soon brought him back to the room, although not yet coherent. I sat with him and we conversed off and on. Let me say that if you want to know someone's true character, sit with them as they come out of anesthesia! Once he said that "they" were bringing someone else in who was hurt worse than he was, as if off a battlefield. He continued "Tell them to take care of him first! I can wait." Then something I did not want to hear, "Oh, look, there are two lights shining over there. They're so beautiful! I'm going to see them." OH NO you're NOT! I was very firm. "No going to any lights! You are staying right here on this earth with me."

Later the doctor came and told us what Russ has already mentioned. It was not a good prognosis. "The damage was already too great." All those years had taken their toll, even *though all the American doctors had felt a strong pulse in his ankle and never looked at a vascular problem.*

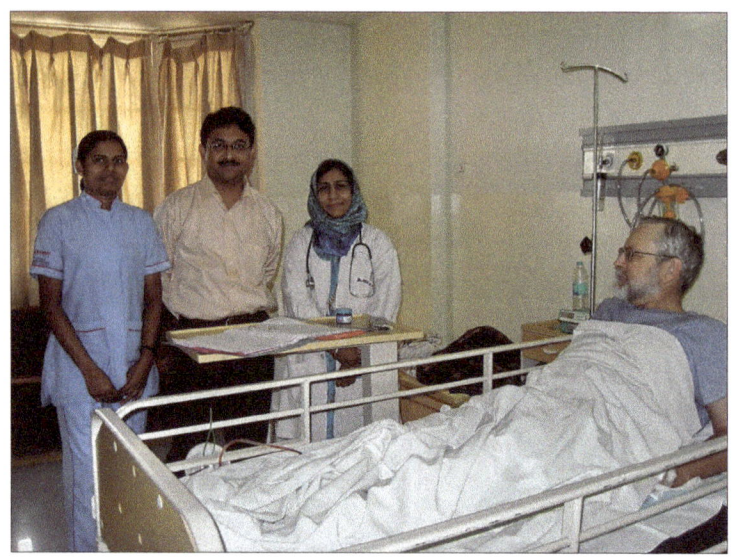

Russ in the hospital, Hyderabad, India

Chapter 10

The Cross Roads of Life

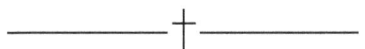

So we finally left India and headed back to the U.S. Before we could leave the hospital all the staff lined up for their tips, from the man who had shaved Russ from head to toe with a straight razor, to the low-caste women who cleaned the bathrooms. Unfortunately, Americans in India are considered about the same as an ATM, since we must certainly be rich. Then, Russ was too tall for the Indian ambulance that was to take him to the airport; they slammed the door on his throbbing foot. Next, the people who pushed his airport wheelchair through the different airports on our way home constantly ran him into the walls of the elevators. His poor foot was quite sore by the time we arrived home. We both were subdued and wondering about the future.

Throughout this time God continued to remind me of the verse in Proverbs 3, and my need to "Trust in the Lord." And unknown to me, those words would one day carry me through the worst years of my life.

From that point on, the health of my legs continued to deteriorate. By November 2010, my left foot and leg were swollen and discolored, and the extreme pain was almost unbearable. I could not even touch the leg without screaming. We had no health insurance, but based on the recommendation of our family physician we went to St Francis Hospital in Tulsa, Oklahoma. To avoid gangrene and save my life, they preceded to remove my left leg below the knee. That is the optimum site so I could walk again with an artificial leg in the future.

It's very difficult losing a leg, both physically and emotionally. It has been my means of mobility for over sixty years. I had hitchhiked across this nation several times back in the 1960's and 70's, hiked over 450 miles of the Appalachian Trail, trudged through the mountains and forests of Alaska, the continental US, and Australia. And after we met and married, much of that time was with my wife, Alice, and now I was traveling around the world.

Adventure was my lifeblood. Risk is a part of who I am. It helped me to dare things for God where others would not go, and do things others would not do. I questioned my future almost every day. What would I do now? How could I continue to serve the Lord?

Because the wound did not heal, eight more surgeries followed to remove dead flesh. There was continual bleeding and excruciating pain for many months. The time was filled with morphine-induced hallucinations. I couldn't think, and at times experienced incredible pain. My arms were stuck full of IVs. Half the time I was trapped in a hospital bed at home as well. I had never known such misery. But I must say that in all this time, my wife lovingly and loyally stood by my side, and changed bloody bandages twice every day.

And I began to cry out to God. "GOD! What is going on? Why is this happening to me?" And in that still small voice, He said, "Don't worry; just remember to Trust in the Lord."

By May 2011 my right foot and leg was also dying. The surgeon removed my right leg below the knee and removed my left leg above the knee in the hope it would finally heal. This time I could not walk away from the hospital bed or wheelchair. I was stuck and feeling helpless, frustrated, and grieving. I wept, doubting I would ever see India again. In the days ahead there continued to be more suffering and pain. We spent our days changing bandages on two huge, bleeding wounds.

I acquired two staph infections in the right stump from the hospital, and two consecutive infections of Clostridium Difficile, a life-threatening mess. But God spared my life, and, finally, my left leg began to heal quickly. My right leg had almost completely healed, but for a small hole that leaked blood continually. As time went by there were more doctors and specialists. It seemed as if this crisis would never end.

And again, I cried out to God. "GOD! Is this the end of my ministry? Will I never return to my beloved India?" And again God reminded me to "Trust in the Lord."

During the many long months, God continued to be with me. I learned to be patient as I endured suffering. At that time I was still living in a fog of drugs, including both Morphine and Fentanyl patches. At one point, the pain was so bad I was taking an intravenous cocktail of Morphine, Dilaudid, Fentanyl, and Oxycodone. With the help of my God, and my loving wife, I was able to leave the drugs behind. It took three months of shaking and sweats, but the Lord gave me the strength to conquer the addiction.

Finally, after eighteen months of constant care, both stumps healed, and for the most part, the more severe pain had receded. Of course, even today, the cut nerve endings and phantom pain is always with me in varying degrees; sharp, real, and permanent. I continue to lose many nights of sleep, and I will be on oxycodone until the day the Lord calls me home. But the Lord is good, and no matter how much "bad" happens, God always gets me to where He wants me to be. All during this time He continued to remind me to "Trust in the Lord."

At one time or another most of us struggle with pain and sorrow. Yet, God's presence is like a warm blanket wrapped around us in the form of a cocoon, protecting and sheltering us, and allowing a deep, inner joy to surface, no matter how crushing the situation appears. During all this time I felt God closer to me than at any time in my life. As all my family and friends showered me with their tireless love, I began to better understand the depth and undeniable beauty of God's love. After all this time I have come to realize that the day will come when I will be healed. Philippians 3:20-21 says that our bodies will be "glorified" in heaven. Glory be to God!

One of the most humbling things about all this was watching my wife, Alice. Each and every day she would get up early in the morning, attend to me, work a 40 hour a week job, feed me, bathe me, change my bandages, and love me even when she was exhausted from a long day at work. And God, himself, walked us through all of this.

Alice: Even from my perspective, although I was not the one directly experiencing the pain of sawn bones and severed nerves, this shared experience was an unreal nightmare. We had come to Oklahoma for a "temporary" job with Russ managing a Storage Unit and U-Haul business. It came complete with an apartment so we could, as we thought, scope out the area and see what the future held for our retirement years.

During Russ' recovery, I was doing all the physical and office work, plus caring for him. The job entailed a lot of work, but that was fine with us. We are no strangers to work:

checking the property constantly for security, disposing of the nasty mattresses and sofas left behind by unscrupulous clients, maintaining the grounds and buildings, cleaning out emptied units, including mice, brown recluse spiders and numerous crickets who had taken up residence there. I also processed leases, chased down delinquent payments, and cooperated with the police who had reason to believe drugs were stashed in a unit. We once reported finding the makings of fake IDs in one unit that was deserted. I oversaw the twice yearly auctions of abandoned unit contents; which became a madhouse due to the TV series that showed hidden treasures discovered in storage areas. I also produced detailed monthly financial reports for the owner, made daily bank runs, hitched up heavy U-Haul trailers and vehicle carriers, and cleaned out the big trucks readying them for the next rental. This often meant wiping up spilled cola and fried chicken bones, and emptying ash trays, sweeping out nails, trash and broken glass from the rear cargo area. Many times I had to fill up emptied fuel tanks of trucks returned in the dark of night, despite signed contracts to the contrary. Russ often commented that if anyone doubted the concept of "total depravity" in humanity, they should take a job renting out U-Hauls and storage units for a week. That would definitely change their outlook!

When Russ had his first amputation, it was evident that it was not going to be a short term recovery. The owner, Mike, graciously transferred the manager's position to me, allowing us to continue to have a paycheck and a place to live. The job was quite a bit longer than 40 hours a week, and sometimes people, not reading their leases, would come to their unit late at night and be unable to leave since the gate automatically locked at 11pm. We would sometimes be awakened by stranded renters who were banging on our windows to be let out.

Russ was virtually helpless most of the time. Not only was he in terrible pain and trying to adjust to a new body, trying to turn over in bed without using his legs, but the morphine clouded his mind. I would come in, between customers in the office, to hear him in conversation with people who did not exist. I had to change bandages two or more times a day, soaked with blood. Thank the Lord, he never got an infection in all that time, despite gaping open wounds, but from the hospital visits. They almost cost him his life.

Our living room looked like a hospital. He could not get into the tiny bathroom, so you can imagine all that meant. I would feed him, turn him over, dispense numerous medications, wash him during the week, and bathe him on the weekends with help from our church. That entailed a Hoyer lift, placing the sling under him, rolling him onto it, and then pumping the hydraulic lift so he could be wheeled into the kitchen area. There, I placed a kiddie pool with his shower chair in the middle. We would lower his naked body down onto the chair, release the sling, and the church deacons would sit on the sofa while I poured water from the sink onto Russ. Clean at last! All this was an arduous task that lasted for many long months.

We used our small Jeep Cherokee for the trips back and forth to Tulsa and St. Francis Hospital, for checkups and surgical debridements. I leveled the back seats, added a foam mattress and sleeping bag, and Russ would sleep most of the way down the 412 Turnpike and into the city. Once, after a debridement of dying tissue, we were almost home when I noticed his sleeping bag was soaked with blood. The surgery had not clotted properly, so off we flew to the Stillwater Medical Center Emergency Room. There he waited and waited, blood dripping from his leg onto the floor while I paced. Thank the Lord, all was eventually taken care of.

It was sickening to see his initial amputation during the follow-up appointments. The staples would be tearing out amid jelly-like dead flesh. Every week or two, we hoped to see things changed, but they did not. Finally, when his other leg obviously need to be amputated, they had to re-do the first one. It just would not heal until the second surgery.

I have to say that Russ never lost his sense of humor and boyish playfulness during all the terrible trials we were enduring. On one of his many re-visits to the 5th Surgical Floor of St. Francis, where the nurses knew him by name, the hospital chaplain, a priest from the Indian State of Kerala came to visit. He was amazed that Russ smiled and greeted him. "How can you still be smiling?" was his question. He gloomily droned on about filling up the sufferings of Christ, but Russ responded with a message of hope. God will get us through this, and I will have artificial legs eventually. The priest shook his head in disbelief. We later wondered what exactly his faith meant to him in hard times.

The long passageway from the hospital to the surgeons' offices sloped downhill. Russ would get at the top in his wheelchair, let out a big "Wheeee!" and freewheel down toward the elevators. Nurses and interns would scatter, laughing and cheering him on. I think it was a delight to them to see someone with a positive attitude despite his circumstances. It was a testimony to our hope in our Lord. Russ also was able to minister to others. Once, coming out of the hospital after yet another surgery, he was waiting for me to bring up the Jeep to the door. A man came and asked him for counsel. He was a diabetic and would soon lose a leg; he needed to know how to deal with it. Russ was able to encourage him with the love of God.

What Russ was unaware of at the time, were the long hours into many a night I spent filling out paperwork to lower our huge financial costs. We want to give God the glory, and thanks to the mercy of the hospital and doctors, and to our church family because we are not sinking in debt.

Praise the Lord!

I would be remiss in not mentioning the tremendous love and support I received from my home church, Hillcrest Baptist. Hillcrest has been the hands and feet of Jesus. We had so many nourishing meals, friendly visits, and ongoing financial aid we never expected or dreamed of from them and faithful friends who have been with us since our days in Alaska. A new set of prosthetic legs are completely paid off as well as the huge medical bills which could have drowned us. They gave me encouragement when the future seemed impossible. Let me tell you when you lose your legs you also lose any dignity you might have.

Slowly, I graduated from the hospital bed to a wheelchair, and finally, in March 2012, to my new titanium legs from Scott Sabolich Prosthetics in Oklahoma City. As awkward, slow, and frustrating as they can be, I can walk again! I use my wheelchair to get into the church. In the beginning I was able to stand and look people in the eye again as we talked, instead of sitting at belt level. Eventually, as I got older, I lost strength and balance. I can still dress and drive while balancing on my legs. I can also walk to the bathroom once again. Everyday things I once took for granted are so precious now, restored by the grace of God.

Chapter 11

Return to India

---+---

It was March, 2012, and the technicians at Sabolich Prosthetics, including the owner, Scott Sabolich, were fitting me for my first set of prosthetic legs. As I was learning to steady myself on my new high-tech "stilts", I told them that God was calling me to return to India in May of 2012. They said "Impossible! You haven't learned to walk yet!" But, Praise be to the Lord, our God is the God of the impossible! By May 3rd, I had returned to Tenali, and gone on to minister in Bangalore. And by June 1st I was preaching in Kolkata.

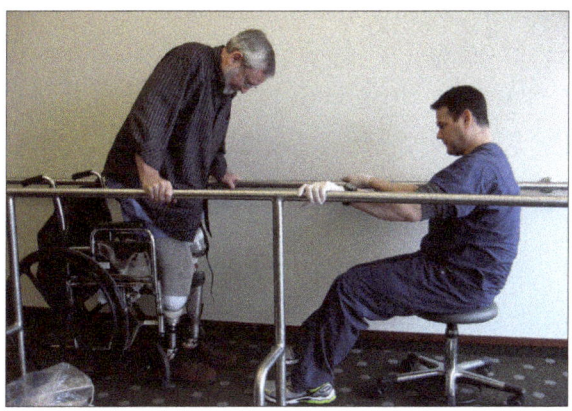

Being fitted for Prosthetic Legs

We were so excited to be back in India for a month doing God's work again! This, in a land which has virtually no accommodations for the handicapped: where all lodgings are 2 or 3 flights of stairs UP, where a sidewalk, if it exists, is usually in disrepair, where doorways have high thresholds to step over, and bathrooms are usually too narrow for easy access, assuming you have a bathroom. It was a difficult but exhilarating trip!

The following year, 2013, I returned to India for 3 months and traveled over 2300 miles preaching and ministering in four different states in India. I trusted in the Lord with all my heart, and He alone opened the path for me, for His glory and honor.

During that trip, amazing things began to happen. I would be ministering in one town or village, and get a phone call from another town. "We would like 'The Man with No Legs' to come preach during village crusades and come to teach our pastors and national missionaries."

Doors opened wide. The rich upper castes were amazed that I would come despite all my difficulties, why? 'Let me tell you about Jesus!' On two flights, as I struggled to get back to Economy Class, an Indian woman in First Class offered me her own seat. We were invited to a Brahmin Caste housetop in an elite neighborhood in Hyderabad to hold a meeting that was obviously heard, via their sound system, by all the surrounding homes. The poor lower castes felt that I understood suffering, which filled their lives as well; so they came to hear what I had to say. The curious came just to gawk, and yet, heard the Gospel of Jesus Christ. Last of all, the lepers, who usually had no fingers or toes, and often no legs, knew I understood their plight. My personal "best" was climbing up the hill, stepping on 50 rock slabs set into the slope, to the Leper Colony above the city of Bangalore, Karnataka, in partnership with Pastor

Babu Prasad. I admit I had to rest on my walker for a while once I reached the top.

Leprosy is a stark reality in India. The government euphemistically declares that the disease is "under control." Perhaps, if you weigh 100,000 new cases every year against 1.5 billion people total. But, lepers total in the millions. Theoretically the disease can be arrested by medication, but not cured; this is supposed to be free to all lepers. But if you know anything about India and its corruption, you would know that few are receiving what they need. I visited a facility in Hyderabad where the prosthetist looked with a sad smile at my prosthetic legs, then showed me the primitive plastic limbs he was barely able to provide to his patients. So many hopeless people were lying on dismal beds, asking me for help. Men, women and children, all afflicted with the Old Testament curse of "Unclean! Unclean!"

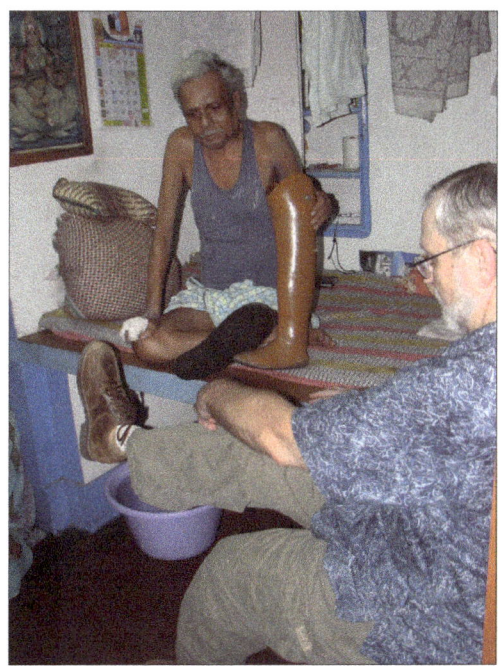

Russ speaking with Leper Amputee

Leprosy is not really very contagious because it requires years of exposure in unsanitary conditions and poor nutrition, yet it still carries a huge social stigma. Lepers are shunned outcasts, and often live in colonies for community and mutual protection. Many villages will not allow them to use the village well for drinking water relegating them to ditch water and disease.

The victims lose feeling in their extremities first, then eyes, legs and other body parts. God's gift of pain is lacking, so they damage their bodies unknowingly. Most have lost all their fingers and toes. Often noses are decayed, and missing legs are common. Sight is lost when they no longer have a blinking reflex to moisten the eyeballs. By this time the disease cannot be hidden, and they suffer the social consequences. They and even the healthy members of their families are no longer welcome in the community.

Alice: I remember the first leper I saw. At an outdoor Gospel Meeting one night, I noticed a woman sitting among the others on the mats, with a little girl on her lap. For some reason, her sari scarf was draped over her face, not just her head for prayer. As she rose at the end of the service, I saw her nose was missing. A leper! I cringed at the thought of her coming up for prayer, not wanting to touch her. She didn't come, just melted away into the crowd. As I returned to our taxi I was convicted. This poor woman needed Christ. I was so wrong in my attitude toward her. We had to leave so I didn't get a second chance. The experience never left me.

Sometime later, we were ministering to a group of lepers, and one was a sad looking lady sitting in the front row near me. Many of her fingers and toes were missing, her face blemished, eyes disfigured and weak. Her frail body barely filled her cheap sari. I was asked to pray for her feet, which were getting worse. She was 61 years old and had had leprosy since the age of 16. As I knelt in front of her, God urged me to TOUCH HER. Jesus did! I put my hands on her feet and prayed. As I stood up, she did also, and I hugged her to me. This was probably the first human touch she had in almost 50 years! She wept and so did I. Jesus came to heal the broken-hearted.

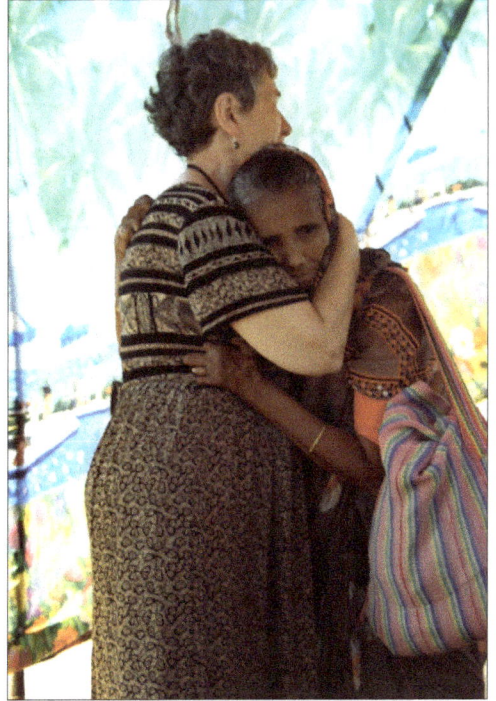

Alice hugs a Leper Woman

Pastor Ravi Sundar of Hyderabad, Andhra Pradesh, had me speak to his church on many occasions to both adults and young people. He also took me to associated churches in rural villages, where people flocked to hear my testimony. At one event, we met young Associate Pastor Victor of Panampally village, who had nearly committed suicide. Early in life, he had been crippled with polio. Hopeless and discouraged, he set fire to himself to end the misery. But it did not end. While he was in the hospital, suffering from extensive burns over 80% of his body, he found the Lord through a visiting pastor who prayed with him. Then he was healed! His Muslim family recognized the miracle and converted to Christianity. We were invited to their little round hut and ate homemade curds and rice with them, washed down with bottles of Sprite, while chickens clucked around our feet.

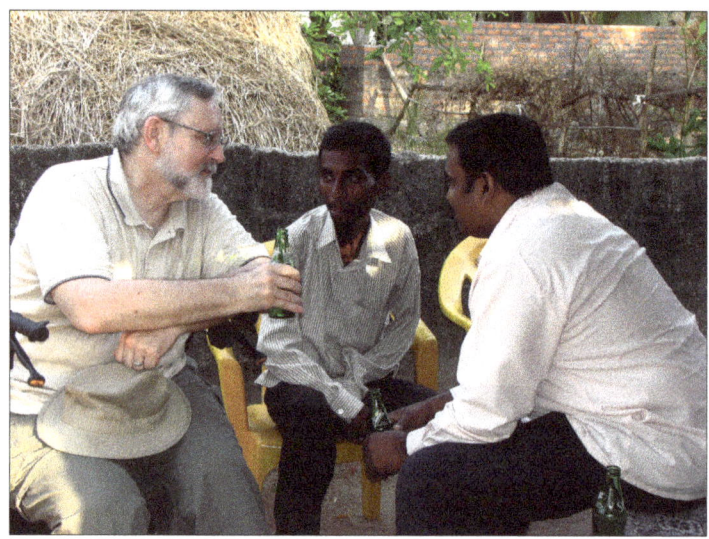

Russ, Victor and Pastor Ravi Sundar

In the many years we traveled to, from, and around India, in primitive villages and not very sanitary cities, it was amazing that we were not constantly sick with dysentery. Alice was sick once, but I never was, even though I ate freely from street vendors and questionable cafés. Part of overseas adventure is eating local foods! The poor always offered their best, sometimes their only food, to us as guests. We could not offend them by refusing even if the outhouse was barely 30 feet from the well.

At another village, we held an open-air Gospel meeting with the requisite stage, bug-attracting lights, and huge speaker system. In India, if speakers are not at full volume, squealing with feedback, reverberating the entire stage and deafening most of the crowd, they are not considered adequate. The crowds began to arrive, seated on plastic tarps spread across the open field. Ladies and children always in front, men back in the shadows. They wanted to see the "Man with No Legs."

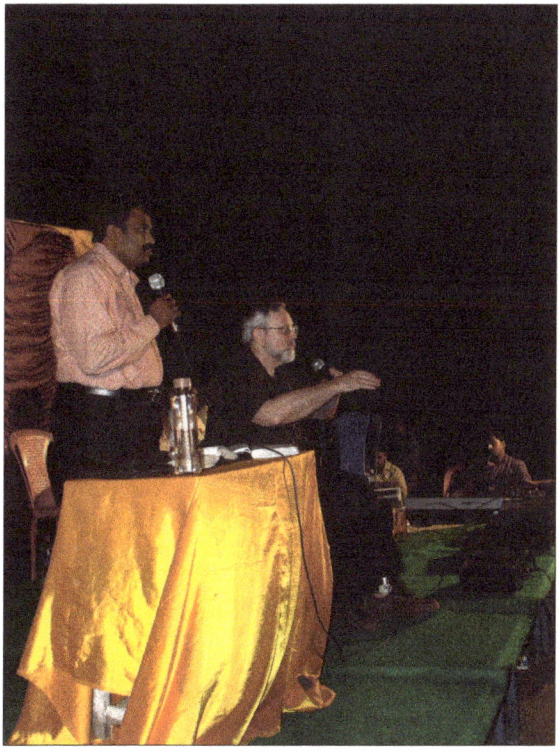

Russ and Pastor Ravi preaching at Outdoor Gospel Meeting

I gave my testimony about how God's grace brought me through my amputations. Then Pastor Ravi preached the Gospel message of sin and the need for repentance. I teased him about our being a "good cop/ bad cop" team; one bringing the love and compassion of God, the other the need for escaping God's justice and wrath. We still have the occasional pleasure of seeing Pastor Ravi since he is associated with the International Christian Assembly of Tulsa, OK and visits them every few years. We sometimes work with their church among the Indian students of Oklahoma State University. They and some of their congregation are our prayer partners and supporters to this day.

In the city of Pithapuram we met with Pastor Samuel Raju and his family. His Grace Baptist Church was the upper level of his modest rental house where I held a widely attended two-day pastors' conference. Alice held a wives' conference under a canvas pavilion on the roof. This was the first ever in that area, and the women were as blessed as their husbands.

We then visited his satellite mission in the village of Kondevaram. The struggling housewives there had to scramble each day, trudging from their little thatched huts to get water from the single government water tap when it was turned on for a few hours. If they missed the timing, their families had no water.

Alice: It's estimated that 40% of a rural Indian woman's day is consumed with obtaining water, carried in metal pots on their shoulders, sometimes for miles. Drinking, cooking, bathing, and laundry are a daily struggle.

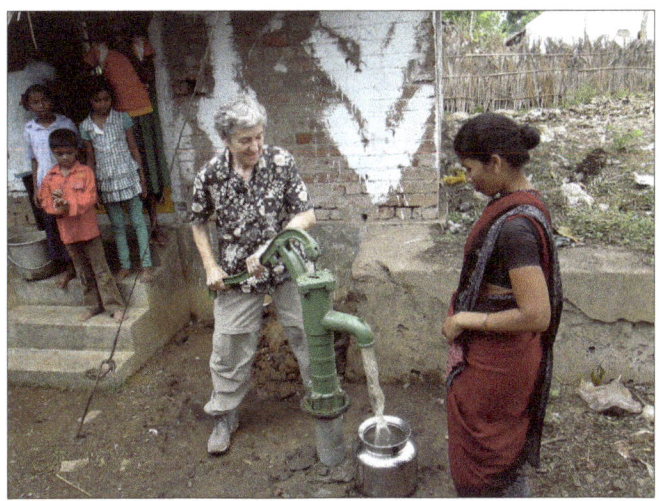

Alice pumps water from new Village Well

Funds for wells had been donated, so one was drilled next to the church using local labor. Water is now available any time, day or night, pure and cold and free. Of course, when Pastor Samuel is there, he interacts with Hindu villagers and presents the Gospel of Christ.

We spent Easter 2013 in Pithapuram at his church, preaching and praising God. Getting up the steep, narrow concrete stairways was worth the struggle to see all the faces lifted in praise and worship. One Lord, One Faith, One Baptism—He is glorified among the nations. And, knowing this was our 10th year of ministry in India, they held a small celebration for us complete with a decorated cake!

During these trips, people were of course curious about my condition. That brought many to listen to the Gospel in churches and outdoor meetings, purely out of inquisitiveness. The adults were usually polite, but the children, especially young boys, just had to know how I walked and what the mechanical legs looked like. So, many a time after the service,

I sat while pulling my pants legs up, showing them the titanium workings as they tapped and looked on in wonder. But another reaction took me by surprise while I was returning to our guest room on a side street in Pithapuram. As I made my awkward way from the wheelchair up the steps through the gate, two little boys stared bug-eyed, then screamed something in Telugu and ran away in terror. I asked our interpreter what in the world was wrong. She laughed and said they had shouted "ROBOT!" I guess they had been watching too many science fiction movies.

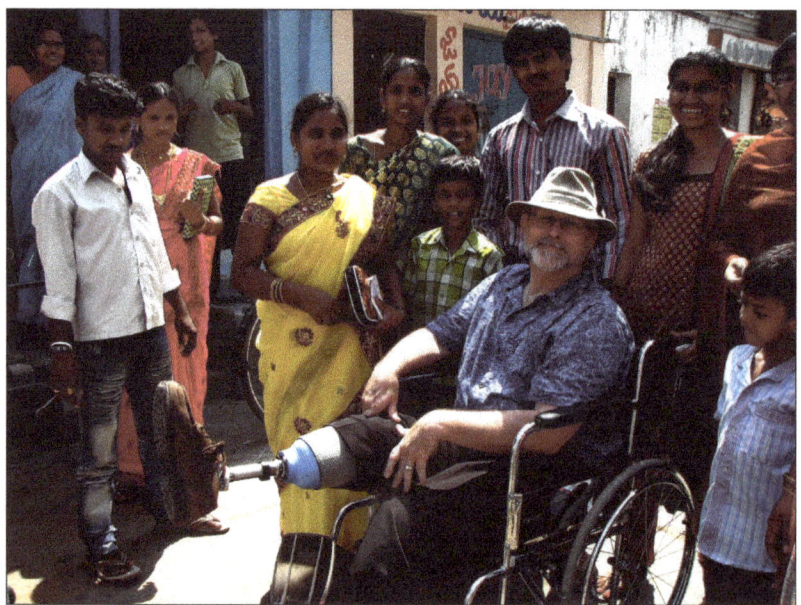

Curious Crowd and The Man with No Legs

We traveled on to the city of Paralakhemundi in the state of Odisha, where the Rajah's palace is a National landmark. This state is where a huge persecution of Christians took place in 2008; thousands of believers fled their homes into the jungles, as houses, churches and schools were burned by angry Hindu mobs. Men were beaten and killed, women, many of them nuns, were raped. Deep scars remain, and many Christians will not return to their former villages for fear of renewed suffering.

Here we partnered with Bihit Parichha, the young and dynamic son of an evangelist. His ministry oversees over two dozen national missionaries in the fishing villages of north Andhra Pradesh, then up into the Eastern Ghat Mountains among the tribal peoples of Orissa. One of his missionaries named John lives in a small lean-to at the end of an apartment building. He and his aged mother have no electricity or running water, yet they work faithfully for the Lord. While we sat on plastic chairs next to his bed in the tiny front room, the neighbors began to fill the doorway wanting to see a Man with No Legs and to request prayer for many illnesses and troubles. My presence brought more seekers to hear the Word of God from John's mouth.

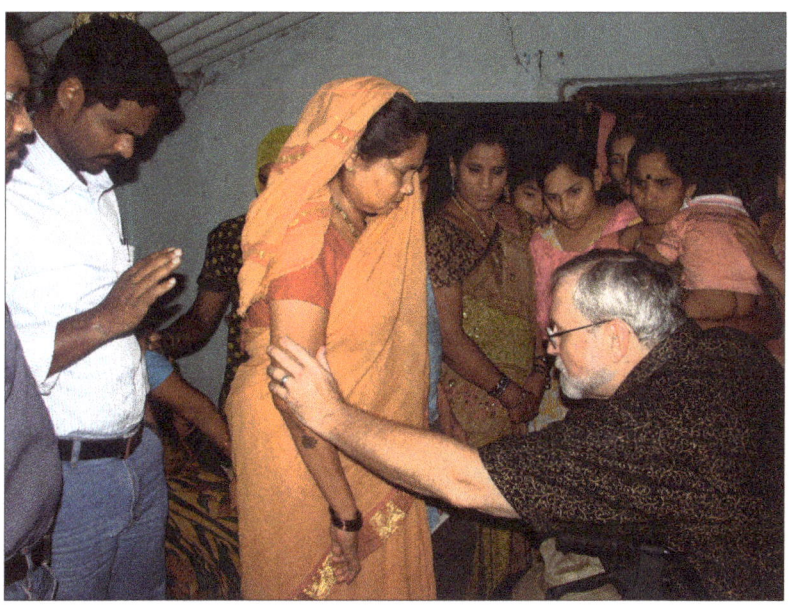

Russ Praying for Villagers

In the fishing villages, I preached in a church with brick side walls, rusting metal roof, and no end wall behind the pulpit area. As poor as some places might be, the Christians are still faithful. Unlike the U.S. where God is often a Sunday thing and life is separate, Hindus incorporate their religion into all aspects of life. When they convert to Christianity, their total commitment transfers. Hymn singing and services are hours long. In some places to get to church, we saw them wading in monsoon rains, with floodwaters halfway up to the knees, take off their sandals, shake out umbrellas at the door, and sit on mats soaking wet for hours for the privilege of worshipping Jesus Christ. At this village, a believing fisherman named Simeon, his assumed Christian name, had recently netted a shark. It was cooked as a specialty for us in a delightful meal.

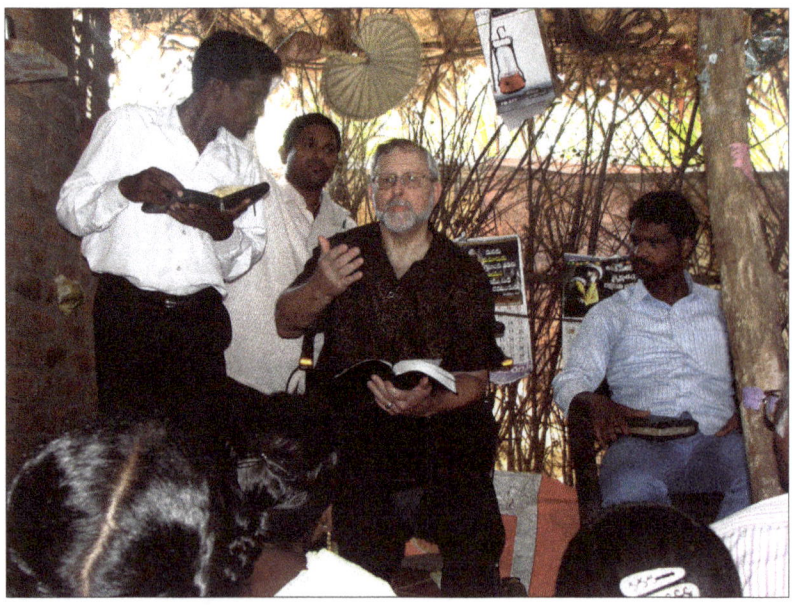

Russ Preaching in a Fishing Village Church

The fishing villages are often the epitome of poverty, although not quite as bad as city slums. The stench of drying fish fills the air, while people walk over sandy layers of dead fish in their bare feet, raking to turn them over toward the blazing sun. Others labor in packing houses for long hours after the gaudily painted boats come into port. The huts in many areas are dilapidated and barely livable. Yet, we saw crowds of laughing boys diving into the water in one harbor, joyful in their youth, waving and showing off to us as we watched from the docks.

It was in this area that I was honored to participate in a group baptism in the surf of the Bay of Bengal. Walking with prosthetic legs through deep beach sand is not for the faint of heart, nor was the hard work afterward as the vehicles became stuck in the same hot sand for over an hour. The service was a highlight of this part of the trip, seeing the joy of new believers committing their lives and their fortunes to Jesus Christ despite a hostile environment.

We in the U.S. have no idea of the cost these men and women are paying for their faith. Loss of jobs and homes, ostracism, beatings, and more are some of the sufferings that are all too common. In fact Bihit received a request to join the search for a national missionary who was working in the hills. His body was found three days later, thrown from the road onto the rocks below.

Then, up into the mountains! On this day, we had to leave in the darkness before 5 am due to a scheduled political demonstration that intended to shut the city down. We were staying in a "lodging" for working class men, complete with brownish sheets and scurrying roaches at no extra charge. The advertised AC worked as long as electricity was available in the city, which varied from day to day and from place to place, usually not when the need is greatest. And, as usual, the bathroom was up several steps, and narrow. Plus it had probably not been cleaned since its installation decades ago. Alice always ran to the nearest kitchen shop for buckets, brushes, and disinfectant when we checked into similar rooms.

The Eastern Ghats have a beauty that rivals travel photographs of Burma and Indonesia. Up and up the road wound. Dawn came slowly and beautifully through the mists. Terraced rice paddies climbed the slopes, surrounded by stone walls. The huts and villages also were picturesquely built of stone. Little streams trickled down the ravines. Looking back, we could see the valleys we left behind, with a backdrop of more blue and distant peaks. The deeper we got into the mountains, the narrower the road became until it was barely more than two wheel tracks.

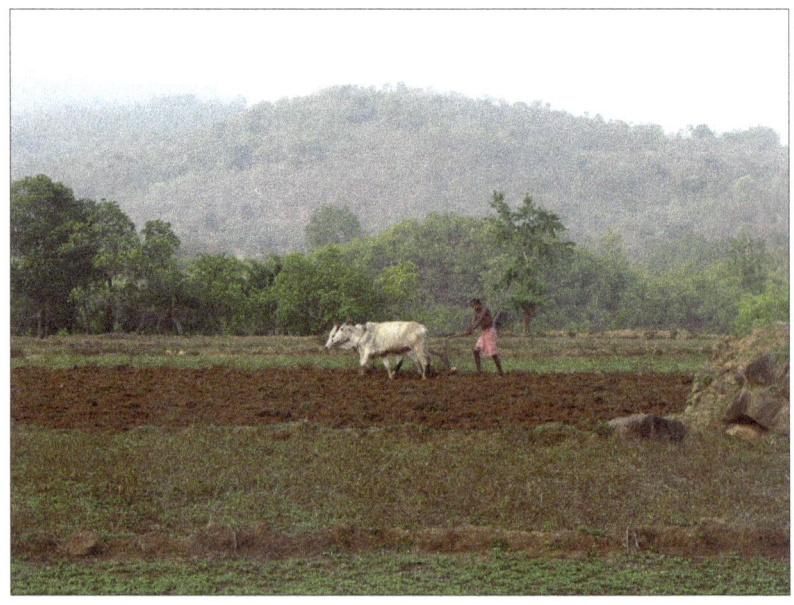

Plowing the Ancient Way, Eastern Ghat Mountains

Finally we arrived at our destination, a large Baptist Church in the village of Puttasingh. Hogs rooted in the ditches, goats wandered in the streets, and women had lined up at the community hand pump across the street. We were given a guest room to rest until time for the service. Unfortunately, kerosene jugs had been stored, and spilled, there, so the odor was overwhelming. The drainage ditch complete with grunting hogs was under the window, with an aroma all its own. And several small boys stood on tiptoe at the window, watching the Man with No Legs taking his legs off. We had to close the only source of ventilation for a bit of privacy. But, as usual, God helped us endure the daily life of another culture, and ministry time came.

Alice held a one-day Conference for the local women, and I preached in the evening service. Among the crowds were tribal peoples, lighter skinned and more East Asian in facial characteristics. Only a few decades ago, they had been uncivilized and uneducated, but were now integrating into society. Most of them had embraced Christianity. We were honored to speak with some of them through an interpreter.

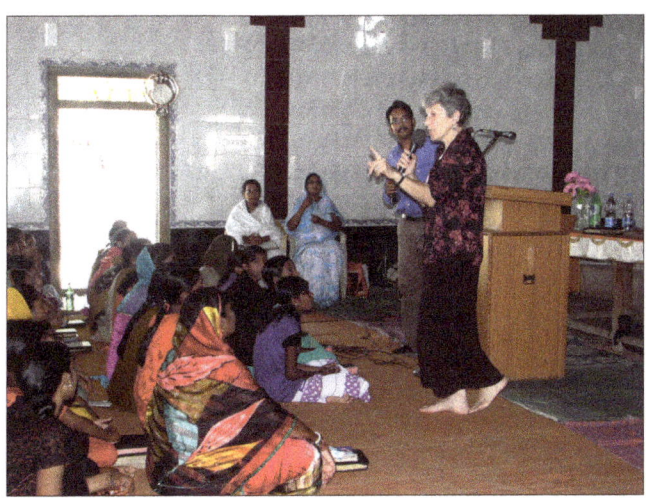

Alice Teaching a Ladies' Conference, Puttasingh, Odisha

On the way back late that night, we noticed that we were not taking the same route. When asked, Bihit casually said this was a longer but easier road to travel. A few hours later, he admitted that driving over the highest ridges was not an option at this hour, Maoist bandits owned the road in the darkness, and had kidnapped some Germans a while back, holding them hostage for many months.

Our ministry time in Orissa came finally to an end. After experiencing the twice-monthly tribal market, we reluctantly said good-bye to Bihit and his small family. His effective ministry became one of the partners of AIM, and we remain in touch with him to this day.

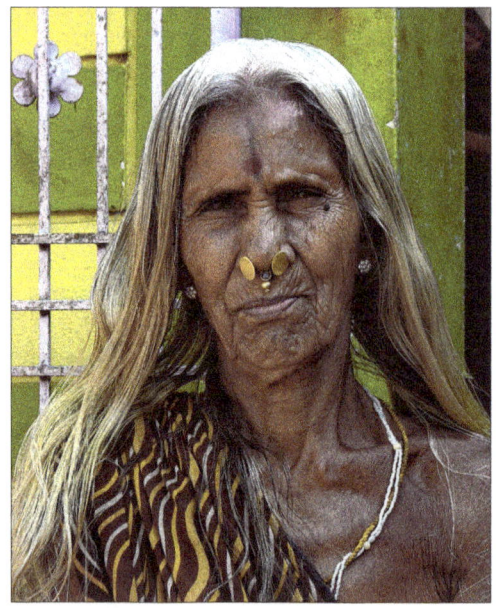

Village Lady, Odisha, India

Alice: The tribal market was one of the cultural highlights of this part of our trip. Women with elaborate gold nose rings sat cross-legged on the ground, offering dried fish, fruits and vegetables of all descriptions, turmeric powder, and other spices weighed on ancient brass scales. Local palm leaf baskets were heaped here and there, including some woven fish traps used in their rice paddies. Crude terra cotta pottery caught my eye. An enterprising vendor was selling flavored ice popsicles from his portable freezer to the hot crowds.

What excited me most was the cattle market! One huge area was thronged with men and animals, some for meat, some for milk, and some for work in a land where the crops are still planted with oxen yoked to wooden plows. Beautiful dark-eyed Jersey cows had wreaths of flowers crowning their curved horns, big Brahma crosses mixed with European stock, and everywhere the men jostled, haggled, and critically appraised the animals, while money and cattle changed hands. This was obviously a huge social event. Some people were dressed in European clothing, some in the more traditional manner of India, some in a mix, whereas just a few decades ago most of the tribals wore little clothing at all. I still remember one man standing alone in the shade with his sleek animal. His one-legged stance was like a National Geographic photo I had seen long ago of a Maori tribesman. The sole of his right foot was resting on his left knee. He was dressed in a loincloth and turban, taking a break while snacking on one of the fruit popsicles. I think for sheer beauty and cultural interest, Orissa was my favorite area of India.

After we flew to Bangalore a few days later, the newspapers were full of a tragic and bloody story. Not far from where we had just been, over the border in the state of Chhattisgarh, an anti-Maoist politician had been travelling along the highway in a convoy with a state police escort through the jungle covered mountains. A young boy tried to warn them away but was ignored. A large group of Maoist rebels ambushed the convoy, killing dozens of people including their enemy, the politician, who did not die a pleasant death. Photos of mangled bodies filled the magazine pages. Who knows from what God may have spared us?

Bangalore in south-central India is a cosmopolitan city in the highlands of Karnataka, probably the cleanest and coolest we experienced. Its tree-shaded streets have fairly orderly traffic which is saying a lot in India. It is also a growing center of technology which brings people from many parts of India, speaking many different state languages. India is one of the most multi-lingual countries in the world. Most speak at least three or four languages plus English.

Here we partnered with Pastor Babu Prasad. He lives in a nicer area of town but God has called him to a poverty-stricken neighborhood. Lepers and single mothers struggle to survive. Women sit in open sheds making incense sticks for pennies a day, barely able to house their children, and often unable to feed them. School is out of reach for most of the poor. Others work long hours as seamstresses in shabby factories. The need is great.

At first, he sat on a street corner singing gospel hymns. People passed by, curious, but kept going. Finally, a lady who was suffering from leprosy became his first convert. From there, a church was born and began to prosper. Today, his vibrant "Mizpah Assembly" is now a landmark on the crowded street, with services in the languages of Kanada, Tamil and Telugu. Their ministry includes the "Nile Project", taking in 50 children from needy local families after school, tutoring and feeding them each weeknight. Once a year the church buys them school uniforms, which are an exorbitant expense for poor families.

On Christmas, a new set of clothes is given each child. We saw many happy faces bent over schoolbooks while we were there, and praised God that He has a future planned for them.

A seven member mission team, from Asia International Mission, flew in from the US to meet us, and we held a four day Vacation Bible School for the neighborhood children. What a wonderful experience! So many enthusiastic children hearing the Gospel, enjoying games and songs, and being fed nourishing meals! Mizpah church members were closely involved in everything and we truly enjoyed working alongside our Christian brothers and sisters.

Later that week, we all went to visit the Leper Colony. It was remote and lonely at the top of a nearby hill overlooking the busy city, and cordoned off by a chain link fence. It is only accessible by walking up the steep slope on 50 huge stone slabs set into the hillside. My personal "best" since losing my legs, was climbing up that hill. I admit I had to rest on my walker for a while once I reached the top.

Families sat in the doorways of their little homes on narrow alleys, and joyfully received us as honored and unexpected visitors. Most of the older patients obviously had no fingers or toes, and other debilitating marks of the disease. While extended family members and children are healthy, the stigma of leprosy prevents them from associating with society as a whole. Separate schools, houses, and culture are the norm. I spent time with one amputee in his home, speaking about the suffering we each experienced and the hope of Christ. It is an honor to know that Pastor Babu's ministry extends to these outcasts that most of the world ignores.

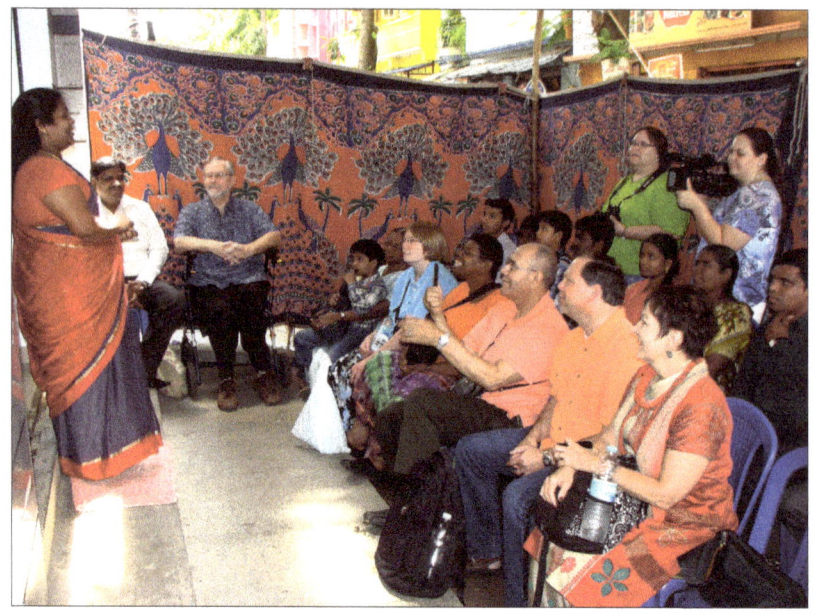

Opening Ceremony, Sunshine Medical Clinic, Bangalore

Pastor Babu's charming wife Suji is a graduate of medical school and an MD. For many years her dream had been to open a clinic near their church in Bangalore, both for the nearby lepers and the poor neighborhood families. By the grace of God, we were able to launch Sunshine Medical Clinic in a moving ceremony. Dr. Suji's eyes were filled with tears as the ribbon was cut, and the first patients, waiting on the street, began to filter in. Her goal is to treat both body and soul. People who can afford to pay are charged, but the poor are treated free. "Freely you have received, freely give…" (Matthew 10:8b)

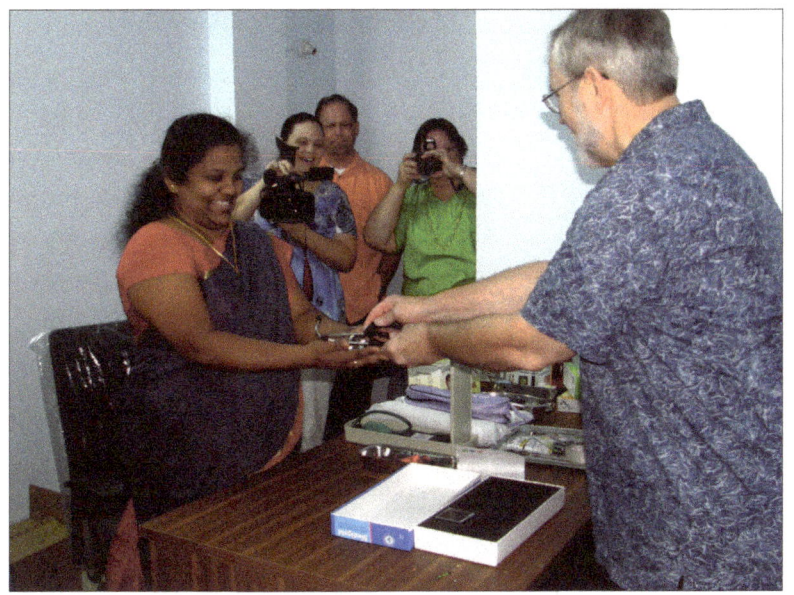
Russ Presents Dr. Suji with a new Stethoscope

Alice: At the close of our stay, the women of Mizpah Assembly honored our Team with a magnificent production of the song "India", complete with a huge silken flag and hauntingly beautiful music. They dressed for the occasion in cream-colored saris, embroidered with gold. It is amazing how different cultures worship in so many different ways, different languages, and different melodies, yet we all follow the same Lord, Jesus Christ! A small foretaste of what the kaleidoscope of heaven will be like!

We then flew to Kolkata, considered the most violent city in south Asia. Cursed by Rudyard Kipling, it was built by the British as a capital for 500,000 residents. Today it and its suburbs house over 8 million, many in unbelievably unhealthy conditions. We were honored to visit the ministry of Mother Teresa, view her grave, and listen to recordings of her Christ-centered sermons. Here we partnered with Paresh Haldar, who conducts ministries in the city slums and also in outlying villages. His primary target is the children, which draws the adults to listen to the Gospel being presented. We and our mission Team from the U.S. stayed in a "real" hotel, and held a VBS in the jungle village of Dihi. Our American friend Pastor Albert May, formerly of Perkins, OK told the stories in his inimitable style, while the women oversaw crafts and games.

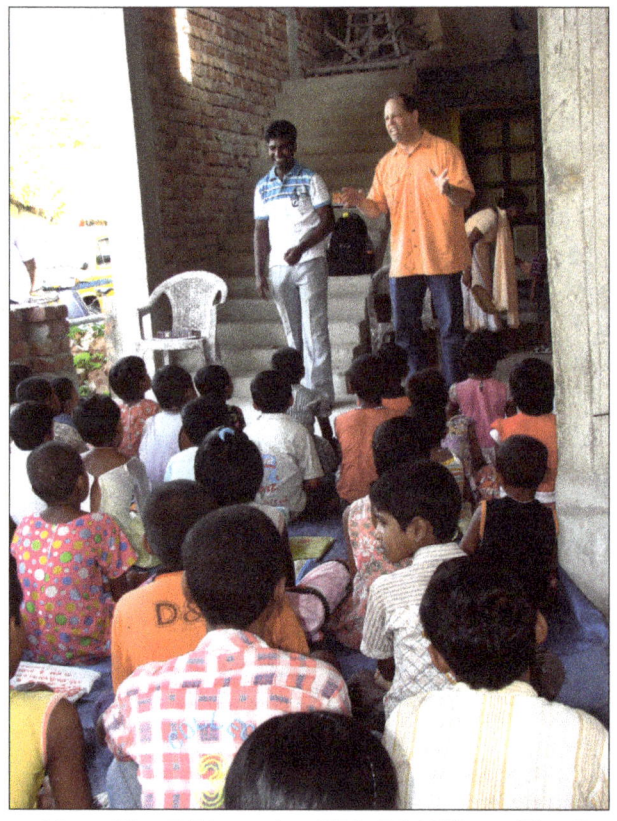

Albert May telling Bible stories, VBS, Dihi Village, West Bengal

To our surprise, the visiting adults, including village elders, insisted on doing the crafts with them! It was amazing to see dignified grown men, sitting on the ground, wearing gold cardboard crowns signifying our heavenly reward for following Christ. And even more surprising, elders from a neighboring village invited us to bring our Vacation Bible School to them and their children as well.

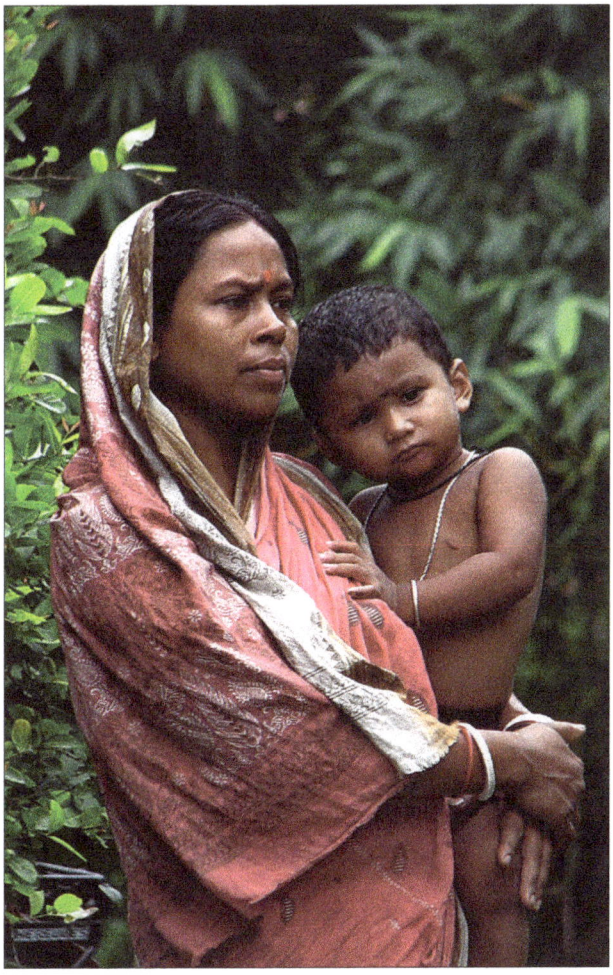

West Bengal Mother and Child watching VBS

Chapter 12

The Times, They Are Changing

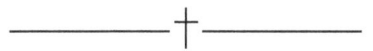

In 2014 and 2015 more surgeries were required as my hands deteriorated due to heavy use transferring from bed to wheelchair, to shower chairs, etc. So, knowing I had many months of recovery, I relinquished the leadership of Asia International Mission to the Board of Directors, who in turn elected Pastor Albert May as the new Executive Director. I was very supportive of their decision and I believed that Albert and his wife would do an excellent job. He and Cindy had a heart for missions and a love for the people of India, as well as being very personable and excellent speakers. They continued to partner with the many ministries who are forging ahead in India among their own people and for the Kingdom of God.

Sadly, a couple of years later, Cindy unexpectedly passed away. Albert has been devastated by the loss of his lifelong wife, ministry partner, and best friend. But, he continues to move forward and we continue to lift him up before God's throne for strength, wisdom and guidance. A new challenge has arisen. After eleven years of ministry, and covering four states, Asia International Mission is no longer allowed into India. Their government has become very nationalistic and anti-Christian, adamant in their desire to make India an exclusively Hindu nation. Many of the individual states had passed anti-conversion laws and even held reconversion ceremonies where Christians were forced to convert back to Hinduism. AIM has since changed its name to World Focus Partners and has redirected their ministry toward Europe where Albert and his friends have worked previously. God will continue to use them to bring glory to His Name in all nations!

Just as I was regaining my strength, the enemy struck again. Alice and I had taken a heart stress test in 2012 and were assured that we were both healthy and functional. In September 2015, just before my birthday, I began having painful episodes which our doctor thought might be acid reflux. The pain would recur every few days and get progressively worse. One time it was so painful I had to pull off the road while driving to let it subside. By this time Alice and I both became very concerned. It happened again early one morning, and Alice called 911. They rushed me to the Stillwater Emergency Room, and my cardiologist, Dr. Poludasu, found a 96% blockage in that old familiar anterior descending artery of my heart, the "Widow Maker." He then transferred me by ambulance to Oklahoma Heart Hospital in Oklahoma City.

There, Dr. Randolph, an expert in the CABG procedure, told me that I had only 3 months to live without open heart surgery. It was a bit of a shock. What about that stress test a few years ago? I had been faithfully taking my daily dose of Plavix for years, so the level had to be reduced before I could go in for a triple bypass. The day finally arrived. Alice and our friend Ann Pardue sat in the family waiting room during the entire procedure, praying and waiting for hourly phone updates from the surgical team.

Alice: About the fourth surgery update, the assisting surgeon said "Everything's going well. We've restarted his heart and..." WHAT! I'm not sure I heard the rest of the sentence. They hadn't mentioned to me that they were going to STOP his heart to work on it!

I awoke slowly over several hours, full of tubes and drains and IVs. The next few days were a bit hazy. Then I came home to another hospital bed and more convalescent gear. I couldn't turn over by myself, and had to hold a teddy bear, provided by the Heart Hospital, tight against my chest whenever I coughed or sneezed. Embarrassing for a grown man to say the least. More long months of recovery, made longer by the fact I had no legs and could not walk like other patients to regain strength. My poor rib cage, which had been sawn apart and stretched open to reach my heart, was aching, and the huge scar down my chest was painful and tender. Fortunately, Alice did not have a full time job to worry about, so she could take care of me with less stress; she did continue painting in her home studio for her art clients. It seemed that my world had closed in once more. But God continued to remind me to "Trust in the Lord..."

He had spared me again and I began to heal and think about a future. The year 2016 found me wondering if my beloved India, its spices and monsoons, rice fields and drainage ditches, beautiful saris and miserable slums, were now a thing of the past. It had been many long, hard plane rides of over 22 hours; many layovers; difficult steps to climb; and all the other trials faced by someone who has limited mobility. I had never regained my balance, so my walking is still awkward and slow. But my mind and heart have always wanted to go to the mission fields for the Kingdom of God. Will I have to resign myself to memories?

Was God finally through with me? Again, His still, small voice echoed in my soul: "Trust in the Lord with all your heart…"

I had filled my life with international ministry at Hillcrest Baptist Church facilitating a Bible study organized by our friend Rosalie Larzalere, with Asian research scholars who came to Stillwater for post-doctoral studies. They came mostly from atheistic cultures, but their intelligent, inquiring minds delved into the truths of God's Word with hunger and curiosity. My co-workers and I saw many come to faith in Christ, and head to their home countries to lead Bible studies among their peers. One entire Vietnamese family was baptized during that time.

Twice a week I post devotionals on my blog called "Life's Journey." I also have the privilege of ministering to people across a broad cultural spectrum and in many countries around the world. Another online ministry has been among the Hmong peoples scattered across the US, mostly refugees from the Vietnam conflict and their descendants. I was introduced to these groups by friends Wayne and Alina Yang from my days at Toccoa Falls College where we shared laughter and Alina's hot egg rolls. I spend many a night answering theological questions and interpreting Biblical passages for people with deep questions about God and life. As a result, we have many friends we have never met face-to-face, friends with a shared faith in our Savior, Jesus Christ. God's Word never returns unto Him void!

Chapter 13

The Caribbean Call

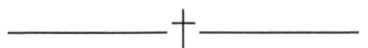

While online, I began to notice Facebook posts by our friends, Pastor Tad Walton and his talented wife Janis, from our past ministry in Idaho. They had decided to become full time missionaries in Gonaives, Haiti. Eben-Ezer Mission Inc. is a Haitian founded and Haitian-run organization helping their own people through education, small business development, agricultural projects and other ventures all based on the Gospel of Jesus Christ. We began to read of their adventures and progress, then started correspondence. Hmmm, was this a possibility, closer than India, yet in a similar spiritual and economic situation?

In February of 2017, Alice and I decided to take a trial trip to Haiti to investigate the mission and pray for God's guidance. While there, I held a two-day Christian Leadership Conference for pastors and community leaders.

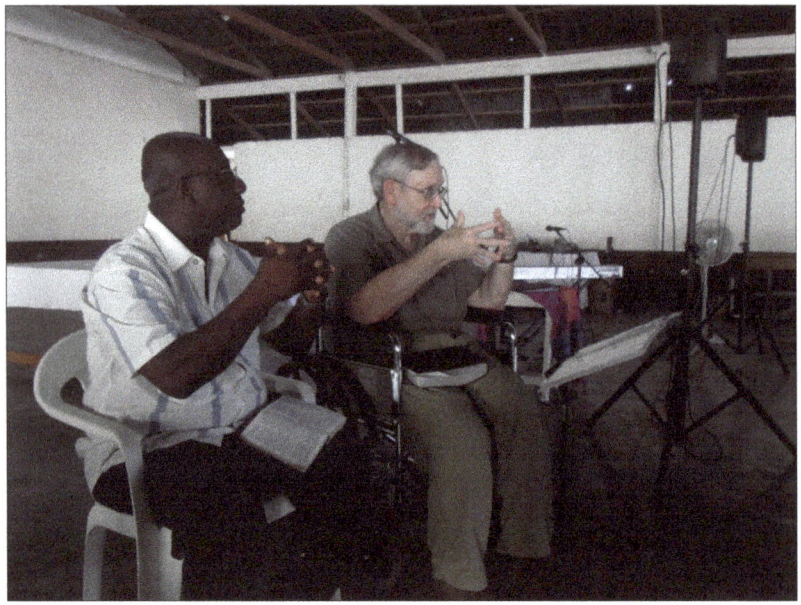

Russ Leading Christian Leadership Conference, Pastor Josué interpreting

Alice held one for the women, attended by a prominent judge. Plus she taught an art class for the children at their *Maison d'Enfants (Children's Home)*. We explored the possibilities and prayed about the future. I was greatly encouraged by the acceptance and response of both the attendees and the mission leadership. Despite my being older and slower, they valued the years of experience I brought with me to pass on to young and old alike. One thing other nations have that is sadly lacking in the US is respect for the older generation and attention paid to their wisdom. Alice and I felt we had found our niche in God's work once again.

We discovered that the mission founder, Pastor Michel Morriset, had for several years been dreaming about a couple of projects that Alice and I "just happened" to have the skills and background to help them develop. So, as I write this, we have been at their satellite Mission in Lacroix, about 15 miles south of Gonaives, for over two years.

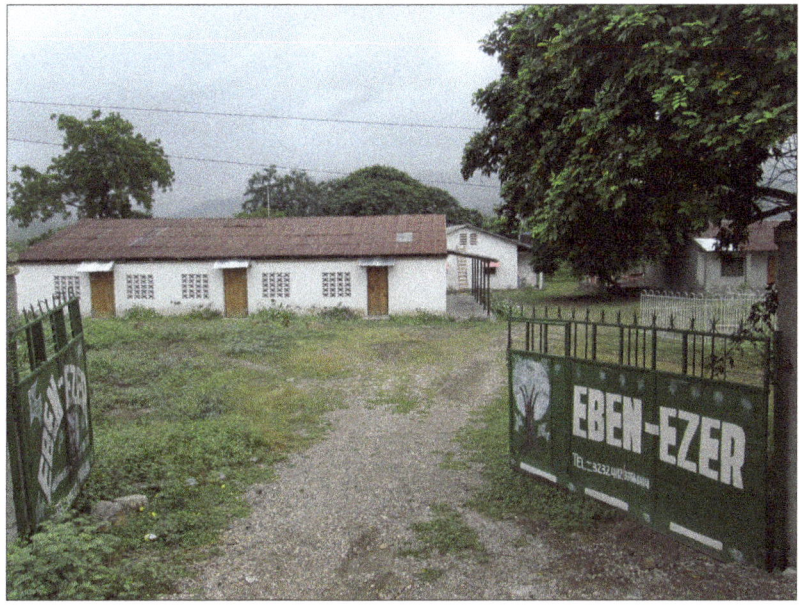

Lacroix Mission

The aging Mission House was barely livable when we arrived in early September of 2017. Little about the house was functional. The heat and humidity were unbearable, no water was available for showers due to an unreliable generator, no power was available for the other necessities of life there, not even cell phone service, and no vehicles were available. No one local spoke English, my laptop was refusing to function, and we were ready to buy return tickets. For the first time in our lives, the enemy had beaten us to exhaustion by constant erosion, day and night, for four long weeks. But, Pastor Josue, our supervisor, hurried to our side and convinced us to stay just a little longer. And by God's grace we started to adapt to off-grid living. Additional solar panels on the roof and the discovery of an internet café we visited once or twice a month in the city of Gonaives helped us tremendously. The additional power enabled us to continue our teaching and preaching work, plus survive the tropical nights with a fan placed at the foot of our mosquito-net draped bed. Since then, we have been able to tap into a new fiber optic cable recently laid from Port Au Prince, the capital city, to nearby Gonaives—this has increased our communication options exponentially. And helped relieve the feeling of isolation in a strange new country where we are in the definite minority.

Roosters crowing in the yard, geckos chirping on our walls at night, and the ever-present neighborhood goats have added a rustic touch to our workplace among the mountains. And those mountains have already sheltered us from the onslaughts of Hurricanes Irma and Maria, breaking the force of the winds which devastated other areas of the Caribbean. The rains were another story but we survived them also. Only a few leaks were evident in our old metal roof, none that fell on our beds.

Alice: Russ doesn't mention the thousands of ants that seem to find every little spatter of cooking oil on the counter even though I wipe it down with Clorox solution. They have fierce stinging, itching bites like tiny wasps, and love to attack my sandaled feet, especially when I go out to hang the laundry. Russ laughs and says they never bother HIS feet; he doesn't HAVE any. He has a total lack of compassion sometimes! They often invade our bed in swarms, scavenging a dead mosquito fallen alongside our mattress, a nightmare to wake us up at 1AM! I admit the Lord has helped me find solutions to these problems, and I too, love this beautiful rural area and its hard-working people.

When I grow weary carrying water from the tiny bathroom sink to the kitchen for cooking and washing, I am reminded by the Lord that all my neighbors have it much harder than I do. In fact, 85% of the world lives like this. Wrinkled old women, local housewives, and even little girls and boys spend many hours carrying 5 gallon buckets of water on their heads, sometimes for miles, to their humble homes.

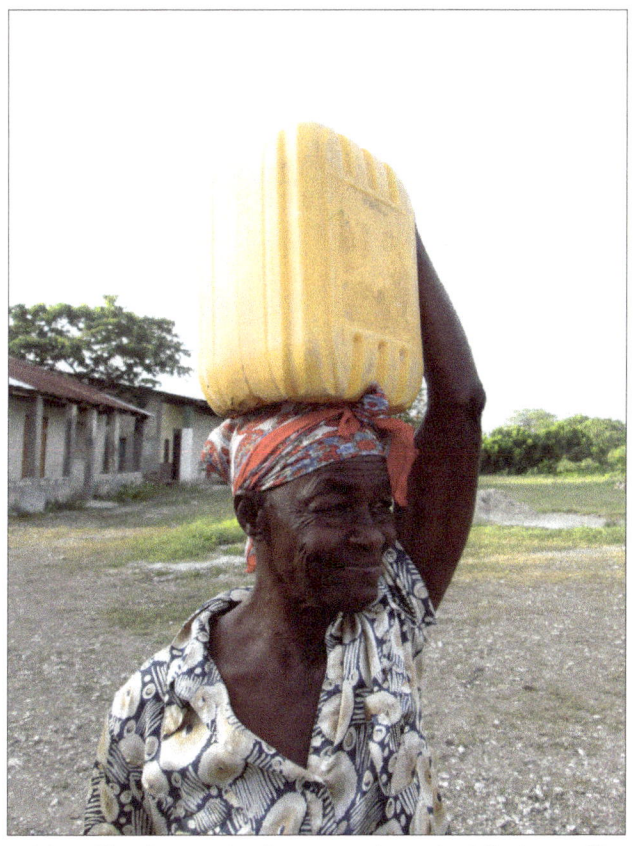

Mezi Charles carries her water from the Mission well

Others might have burros to help them lug 4 containers at a time in panniers. Nevertheless, the daily struggle for water is a reality of life in the Third World. Ladies carry huge baskets of sticks, also on their heads, scrounged from the roadside brush to cook their meals. Others make homemade charcoal from spindly trees for themselves and for sale to others. Life is not easy. Haiti is the poorest country in the Western Hemisphere.

On my morning walk, I've been greeting everyone with "Bonjou!" Most are on their pre-dawn trek to work in the fields or sell produce in the town markets, and return my greeting with big friendly smiles. Kreyol is becoming more familiar to me, and they love the fact I try to speak their language.

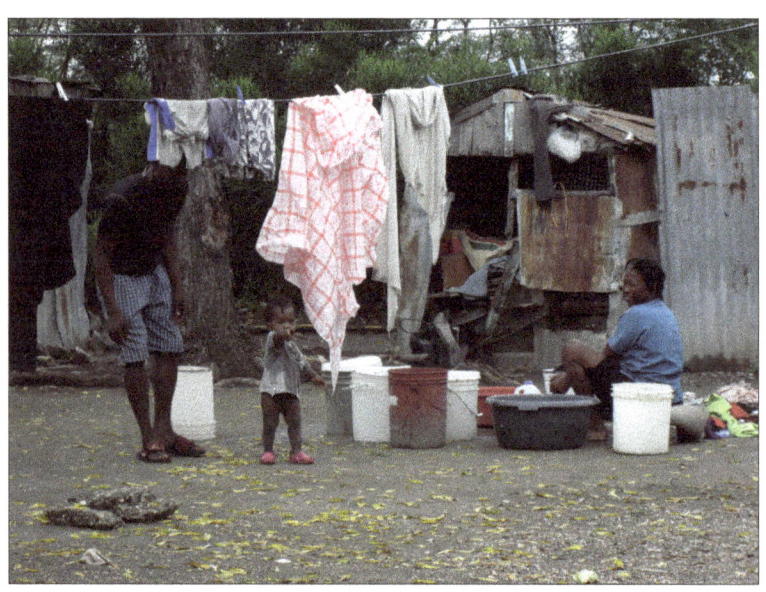

Our Neighbors on Laundry Day

Haiti has a long history of suffering. Born in cruel slavery, it became the first black republic in the world. Liberty was first proclaimed in 1804 in the city of Gonaives, so it has tremendous historical significance. Bloodshed and revenge marked the passing years; greed and corruption at the highest levels continue to oppress the people. Other countries have not really helped the root problems despite huge donations. The funds are often misused and squandered, never reaching the common people. Add devastating earthquakes and desolation by frequent hurricanes to the mix, and you can understand the air of resignation and fatalism that sometimes hinders progress. Yet the people of Haiti are resilient survivors.

Russ and I are working with Eben-Ezer Mission and their Universite' Chretien Haitien (Christian University of Haiti) to educate a new generation with Christian values and the knowledge to think ahead both for themselves and for their country. These students have a chance to change Haiti and the world, with the help of Almighty God. We want to help in any way we can!

I have been helping to develop a Conference and Training Center at the Lacroix Mission which has already hosted a Women's Retreat for large groups from Gonaives, and several pastors' conferences for men from the surrounding towns and villages deep in the mountains. Our first began in the Conference Center building, but the generator broke down, again, and we moved out under the spreading branches of a stately Flamboyant tree. It was a blessed time, followed by a lively question and answer session. I have taken to heart Romans 10:14 which says, "How, then, can they call on the one they have not believed in? And how can they believe in the one of whom they have not heard? And how can they hear without someone preaching to them?" Through these verses God has shown me that they are all hungry for His Word, and I teach the Word to all who will listen at every opportunity. I have preached often at the little rural Lacroix church; and at times, in the church on the main campus of the mission. Both are under the leadership of Pastor Josue Jean. He is the Vice President of Eben-Ezer Mission and someone we have come to love as a brother.

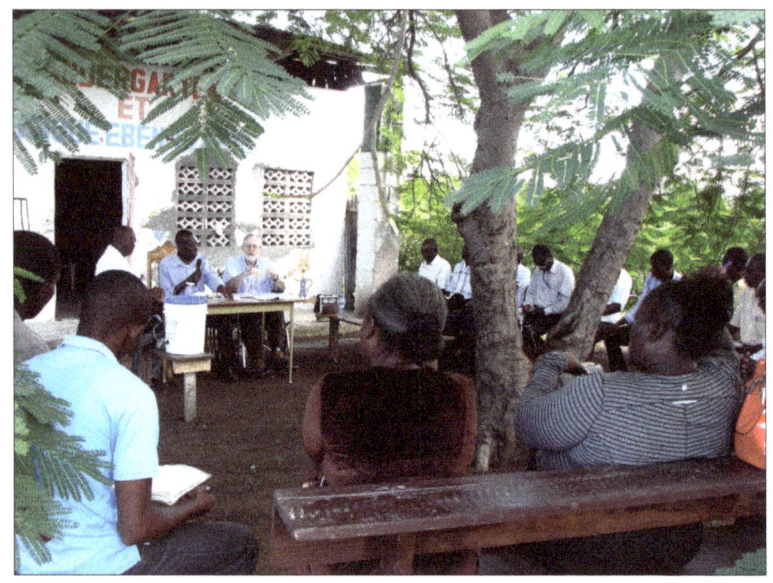

Russ Teaching a Pastors' Conference under a Flamboyant Tree

During our work in Lacroix and Gonaives, Haiti, many generous people have begun to see the vision and future impact of Eben-Ezer Mission. Donations came in for a Solar Power system for the Lacroix Conference Center, so we don't have to worry about frequent generator breakdowns. It now serves the center, the new commercial kitchen also funded by Christian partners, and the two resident families. Frantzcy and Esther Serat are running the nearby Pacot School and the new Lacroix Clinic, respectively. Esther is a nurse; Frantzcy, a tall and impressive young man also provides security for this satellite mission. And, the Fleurvil family, who keep the grounds, do the cooking, cleaning, and generally help where needed.

Alice: Madame Lucsen, as Wiseline [Weez-leen] Fleurvil is called, is an amazing woman. Energetic and enterprising, she knows so much about local herbs and wild plants. I often see her gathering mushrooms after the rains, and other greens from the weeds around the compound. Her husband is currently in Brazil, looking for employment, since there is nothing available in Haiti. (More about this national crisis later) Her cheerful, hardworking daughter Wideline [Weed-leen] does our laundry by hand a few days a week, since this is getting a bit difficult for me. Wideline uses her pay to finish her neglected high-schooling that was abandoned due to lack of funds for tuition, books and uniform.

Madame Lucsen also has her little fast food business on the highway in front of the Mission wall. Let me explain: Other than passing trucks, public buses and a few motorbikes, the local traffic consists mostly of tap-taps, compact diesel pickups fitted with colorful roofs and bench seats along the sides of their beds. People flag them down and for a few Haitian "gourdes," hitch a ride to market, to town, to school, to wherever. Lacroix Mission is at the corner of the National Highway and a main road coming down from the nearby mountains. As soon as it is light enough to see, men and women are up along the Highway ready for market day. The tap-taps roll to an oil-smoking stop, people clamber in, the goods are tied on top of the mountain of freight already teetering there, and off they chug to their destinations. Whenever anyone wants to stop, they "tap-tap" on the side of the vehicle to signal the driver, hence the name.

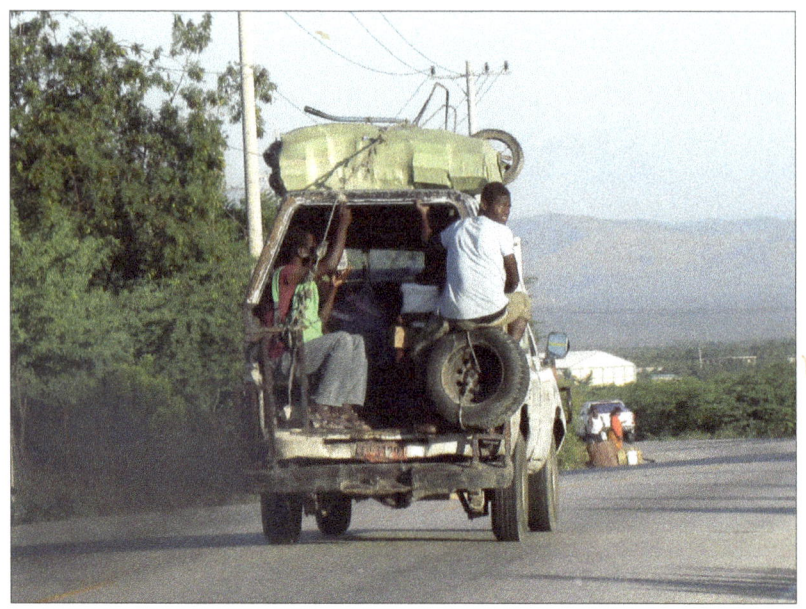

Overloaded TapTap

Anyway, since the tap-taps consider this a stopping place, Madame Lucsen is ready with a huge wok-like pot of hot oil heating over a charcoal or stick fire. She has made a tasty dough with some amazing spice flavors, which she scoops by huge spoonfuls into the hot oil. In a few minutes, out comes a greasy, crispy, delicious "marinad" which costs the TapTap passengers five gourdes (about 10 cents.) She will also top it with homemade "pikle" a kind of super spicy Haitian coleslaw. Then, as a side, she has flattened pieces of fried "banan" (plantain), or maybe hot dogs or fried dried fish now and then, a great idea for four hours work in the morning. Extra cash comes in handy with a houseful of teenagers plus a little 2 year old! We limit ourselves to two "marinad" a week so we don't gain too much weight!

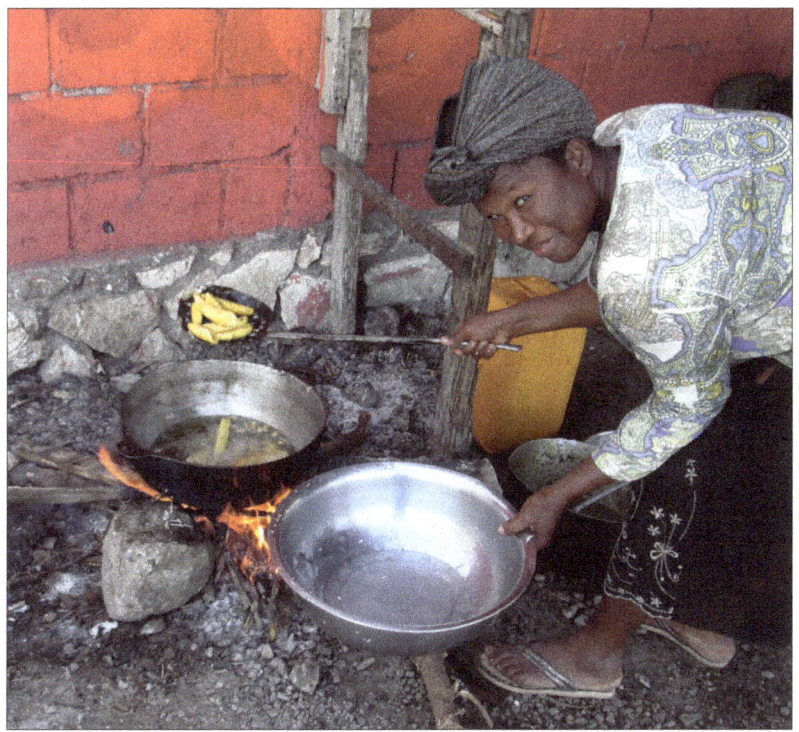
Madame Lucsen's Fast Food Enterprise

Lacroix Mission has several important assets. First, its 20 acres on the main National Highway between the capital of Port Au Prince and the nearby city center of Gonaives. Second, it has a deep 200ft well with pure water pumped up through the gravel and sand by an aging generator into barrels, the high tank alongside the mission house, and another huge community tank near the highway. Each morning we have dozens of local people coming to fill their five gallon buckets with pure, refreshing water. Balancing them on their heads, they go to their little houses with enough for cooking, laundry, cleaning, showers and all the other needs of life.

Another major necessity was adding two large public latrines; not only is pure water a major need in Haiti, but sanitation is usually lacking, causing disease which occasionally escalates into cholera epidemics. We were blessed by a generous couple who donated enough to build these urgent facilities. Finally, the need for electricity was great. It gets very hot in the summer time. We were again blessed with gifts to provide enough solar power equipment to provide for fans and lights in all the buildings on the property. Now the Conference Center can host up to 100 people, feed them, and care for their hygiene too.

Alice: Another national disgrace is the Haitian Diaspora. There is almost no industry in Haiti and consequently jobs are virtually non-existent. Men, especially the younger more ambitious ones, leave to seek paying work in other countries. Since Canada and the US have squelched most opportunities, the men have turned to the nearby Dominican Republic, and to Brazil, Chile, and other places to seek employment. The theory is to land a job, send home money to the waiting family, and return when savings have built up. Unfortunately this theory usually crumbles quickly. Haitians are treated like slaves with low pay and hard labor. Living costs are higher than imagined. Women of dubious virtue provide temptation to lonely workers far from home. Soon the money, if it ever came, ceases, and thousands of women are left alone with hungry children to feed. With no source of income most never hear from their men again.

Even in little rural Lacroix, as in many Haitian cities, women wring their hands and seek solutions. There is no welfare system. Some fall into prostitution, grasping for any way to make a few pennies. Others allow drifting men, often with other families, to "stay for a while" during a temporary job that contributes some cash to the household. Soon the woman has another child on the way and gets abandoned again. Frankly, many of the children in Haitian orphanages are victims of this cycle. Pastor Josue sees much of this in the ministry and has devised plans.

First, he envisions Vocational Training in the Conference Center. Already, five young men are learning to install solar electricity, while helping the technician who was working there. As another example, a woman in desperate straits came to Pastor Josue for counseling. Her husband was working in the Dominican. When the husband returned for a visit, the Pastor had a meeting with him and asked him his occupation. "Carpenter." Are you a good one? "Yes...but I have no tools so I have to work for others." Boss LucSon was given a test job. When it was obvious that he was good, Pastor Josue purchased tools for him, stipulating that he had to stay home with his family. Now, Boss LucSon has more work than he can handle. He built a new ceiling in our mission house bedroom to replace the sagging, broken mess that rained dust and rat droppings on our heads when we first arrived. It is a work of art! Future plans depend on obtaining experienced tradesmen who are willing to share their knowledge with the next generation. Anyone in the US who is willing to spend a few weeks or months training young people is hereby invited to contact us! The chance to change lives and eventually, a culture, is yours!

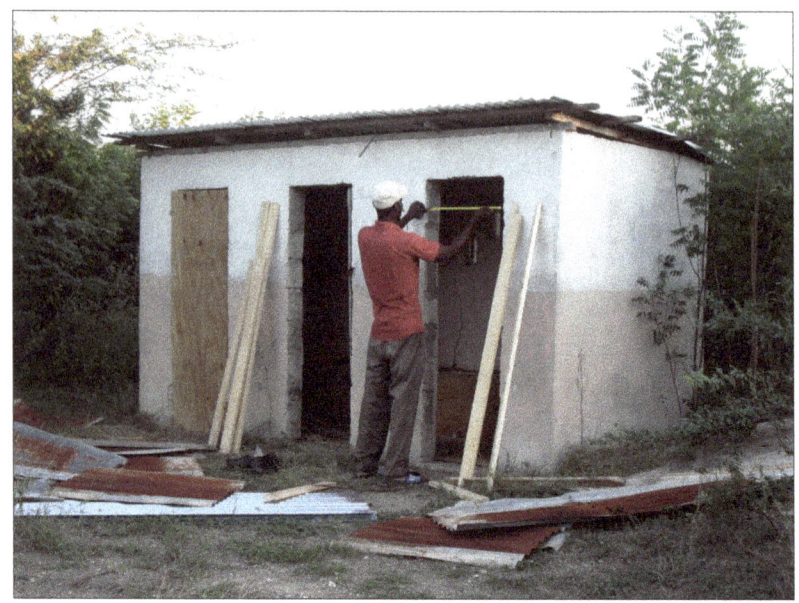

Boss LucSon hard at work

I personally have been a professional wildlife and sporting dog artist for 43 years, making my living by selling my work to clients around the world. I began when it was difficult for a woman to break into a man's domain, but I soon earned the respect of sportsmen because I knew my subjects and worked unceasingly to improve my God-given talent. Now in my seventh decade, I felt it was time to pass this knowledge of painting and sales experience on to a new generation. What better place than Haiti, where opportunity is so hard to come by? It is amazing how God uses the tapestry of our lives to weave into a future He has already planned!

The Christian University of Haiti gave me an old building to renovate by fundraising; I thank God and all the generous people who helped us get a new roof, solar electrical system, and a real bathroom for my avid and energetic students.

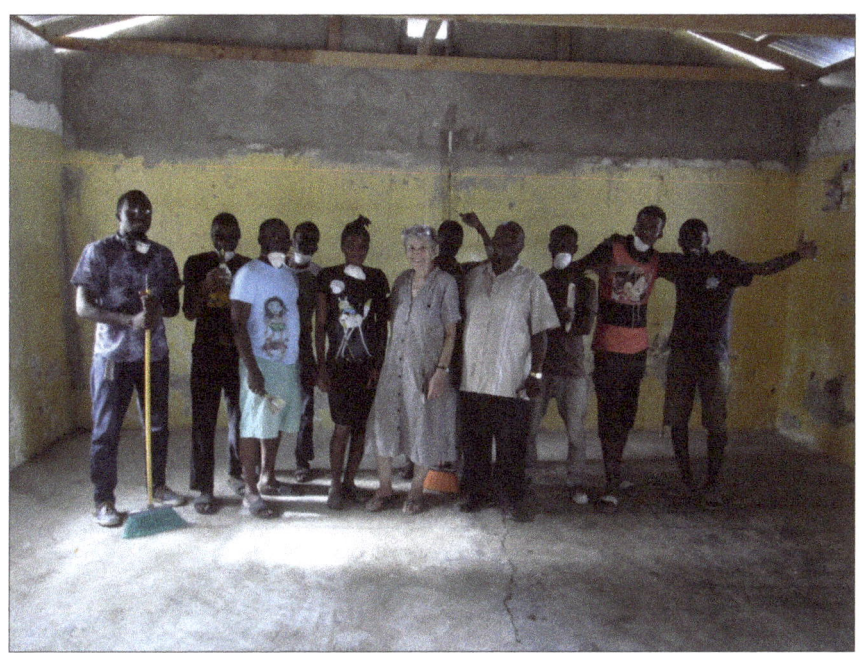

Alice's Art Students Renovating old Building

The students formed the "New Generation Artists Association" to promote their venture under the mission's umbrella. I am helping to mentor them not only in Color Theory and painting techniques, but in how to sell work to the public. It is not easy since I don't know Haitian culture very well, but we are all learning together. My vision is to help revive fine art in Haiti. At one time during the 1960's it was world-renowned and I believe can once again provide income for my gifted young people! I love them like family and pray for them constantly. They are the ones who will change their country!

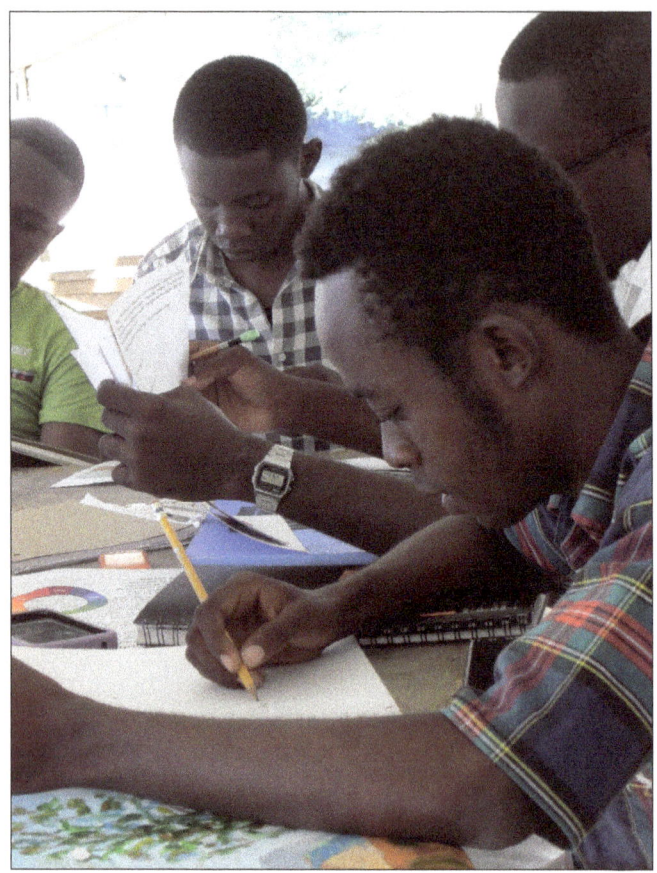

Art Students at Class

Another crucial need in the country is private security protection. Every bank and gas station has armed guards including most supermarkets. In a country where the average person lives on less than $2 per day, hunger becomes rationalization for rampant theft, especially if your children are crying. Even nominal Christians feel God will look the other way if they are taking what they need/want from the "rich" and that includes struggling mission organizations who are trying desperately to better the lives of the same people. Pastor Michel tries to explain that the few *gourdes* that a valuable item is pawned for is not worth the damage caused to the work his mission is doing for the community. Things still disappear if not locked down, but fortunately our Lacroix Mission has not experienced any loss of goods or equipment, besides a few spindly trees chopped down for local firewood while we were not looking. Add the frequent outbreaks of political unrest and an urgent problem is obvious.

Pastor Michel's vision was to develop a Christian Security Team to monitor and protect all visitors, mission staff and personnel, and all assets at the four locations. Eben-Ezer Mission is made up of three facilities in Gonaives, and one in Lacroix. There are 4500 acres on the outskirts of the city where they have constructed three schools, a Christian University, two elementary schools, their large downtown Eben-Ezer School and College, which they call high school, the hospital across the highway from the main property, and the twenty acre Lacroix mission located about fifteen miles south of Gonaives. In Lacroix they have a conference center and church. My years in the military and in private security gave me the needed experience to be able to set up training schools. Instructing recruits fit his vision perfectly. As Alice has said many times, it is amazing how God uses our life experiences for His glory in ways we never dreamed!

I suggested that we start with a small team of six, specifying that we wanted professing Christians who had finished at least 12th Grade and had references from their pastors. Pastor Michel and Pastor Josue convinced me to accept another six; then suddenly it escalated to nineteen young men arriving on a Sunday afternoon, laying out their blankets on the Conference Center floor, and gathering for a beans and rice dinner cooked by Madame Lucsen and Madame Josue, our Pastor's wife.

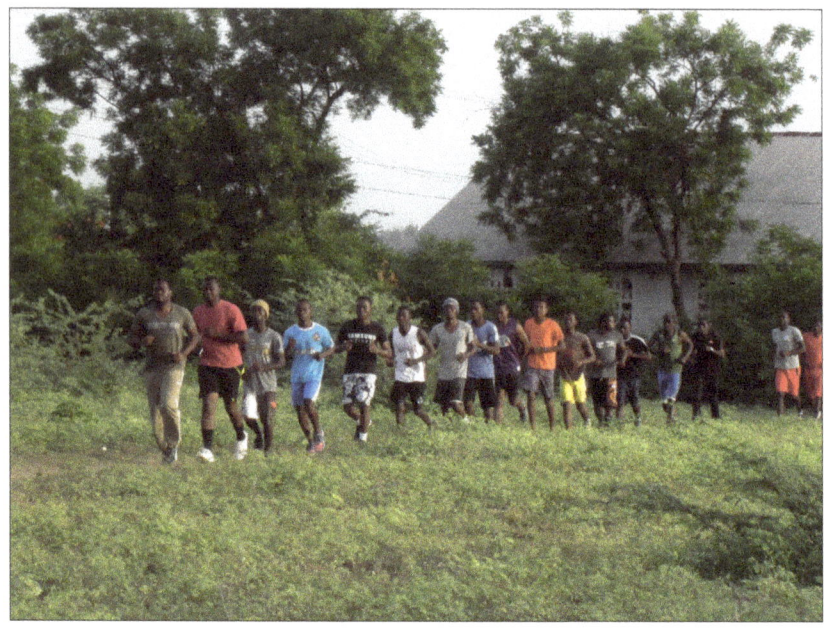

Johnson Alexis leading Russ' Security Recruits

We began each morning before daybreak with my shrill coach's whistle. My right-hand man, Johnson Alexis led them in running two miles to the church and back; soon some of the young men began a Kreyol chant roughly translated "Protect and Serve!" Then rigorous physical training exercises which caused some groans as lightly-used muscles came into play. Next were the classroom subjects on ethics, policies and procedures taught by myself through a translator in the conference center followed by basic First Aid. We then discussed the six levels of the Force Continuum with techniques of self-defense following that. The week was wrapped up with a three hour lecture on Haitian law by a well-known and respected district attorney delineating the difference between security officers and police officers. The young men came to respect me and my knowledge, even though I taught from a wheelchair, because they could understand the value of the training. They organized their own final ceremony on graduation day to display their new skills to Pastor Michel and other dignitaries and received their graduation certificates.

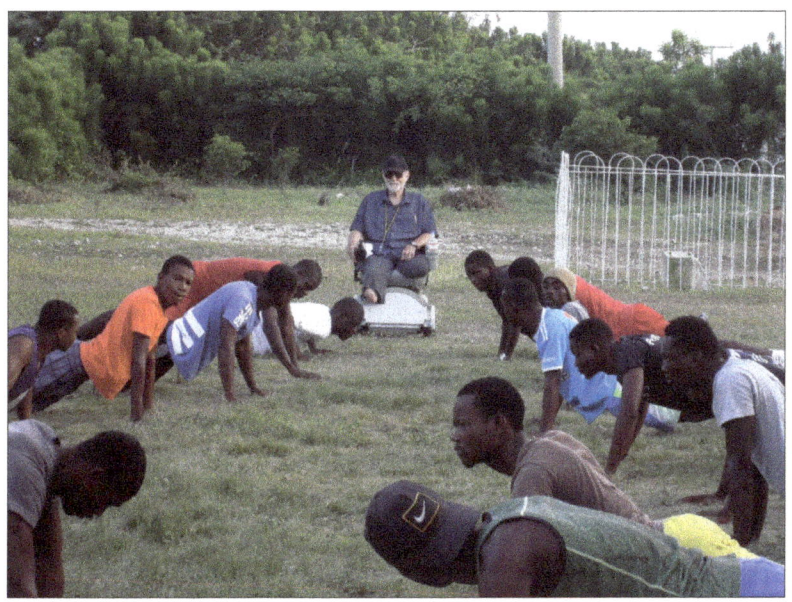

Russ Training the Security Team

I often regretted not having a son to pass down so many of my rich life experiences, but these young men filled that niche. And I had the privilege of seeing some of them become followers of the Lord Jesus Christ. Five of the young men had come from a Catholic background in Gonaives and did not have a solid biblical understanding of the atonement and the meaning of the death, burial, and resurrection of Christ. I brought the devotional after supper each night and Pastor Josue said a few closing words and then a time of prayer. The five men began to ask questions about salvation, having believed that church attendance was all they needed. They also did not see a difference between their friends' lives and the lives of unbelievers. The evening ended with professions of faith and joyful hymn singing. And as scripture tells us, "As the rain and the snow come down from heaven, and do not return to it without watering the earth and making it bud and flourish, so that it yields seed for the sower and bread for the eater, so is my word that goes out from my mouth: It will not return to me empty, but will accomplish what I desire and achieve the purpose for which I sent it." (Isaiah 55:10-11) I always stressed that these recruits should be God's Elite Team, not following the usual Haitian image of a slouching 'gangsta' type security guard who steals from employers, harasses local people, and goes over the fence at night to be with prostitutes. God wants men to follow Him with all their youth and strength! My team of recruits caught that vision and I rejoice in the Lord. Once we receive our official licensing permits from the Haitian government, they will be ready to go.

Many of the things I took for granted for almost 70 years have once again become a reality. I confess I get embarrassed when people applaud my progress, but it also brings tears to my eyes to know that they have prayed and encouraged me each step of the way as I continue to move forward in God's calling. I admit the renewed journey has just begun, and I am still learning something new each and every day. We are prayerfully considering taking a new step in our approach, forming another new mission organization that will not only raise desperately needed funds for the vital work in Haiti, but send other younger people to work there, and elsewhere around the globe, as the time approaches when I cannot physically continue. But I am determined that I will serve the Lord wherever He has called me, and to do whatever He wants done. I may appear old and slow now, but in all that I do, I pray that God will be glorified.

Many times throughout this ordeal, Alice and I, and our church family have asked God for a miraculous healing. But in 2 Corinthians 12:9-10, the Lord reminded me that, "My grace is sufficient for you, for my power is made perfect in weakness. Therefore I will boast all the more gladly about my weaknesses, so that Christ's power may rest on me. That is why, for Christ's sake, I delight in weaknesses, in insults, in hardships, in persecutions, in difficulties. For when I am weak, then I am strong." And as Paul said in Philippians 4:13, "I can do everything through him who gives me strength."

My message is that we WILL have suffering when we follow Christ. Satan will try to discourage us and prevent the Gospel from reaching lost souls. But God will strengthen us through suffering. He will use it to give us a testimony of His grace and mercy, and He will bless us as we continue to endure to the end. His work, His kingdom IS the purpose of our lives!

God has been with me since the beginning. He still has a purpose for my life, as broken as it may be. He used this situation to take away my independence so that I would depend on Him alone, and in Him alone do I trust. And every day I thank Him, as Alice and I make every effort to live our lives in a way that would honor God.

May His Name be glorified!

"Water encompassed me to the point of death. The great deep engulfed me, Weeds were wrapped around my head. I descended to the roots of the mountains. The earth with its bars was around me forever, But Thou hast brought up my life from the pit, O LORD my God. While I was fainting away, I remembered the LORD; and my prayer came to Thee, Into Thy holy temple. Those who regard vain idols forsake their faithfulness, but I will sacrifice to Thee with the voice of thanksgiving. That which I have vowed I will pay. Salvation is from the LORD." (Jonah 2:5-9, NASB)

Alice: As this goes to press, Russ and I are currently back in the US for medical needs. He has been suffering extreme pain on his right hand which has prevented his ability to work and his mobility, due to severe carpal tunnel syndrome as well as failure of the 2014-15 surgeries. Surgery on his right hand was done on June 14, 2019 and he is currently working with a hand specialist in physical therapy twice a week. The Lord is healing him and progress is obvious. We are confident that our future will continue in service for His Kingdom.

Riots and political conflict began again in earnest shortly before we left Haiti, spreading from Port Au Prince to several other urban centers. Most missionaries left the country, although Tad and Janis Walton have since returned, confident that Eben-Ezer Mission will not be the target of violence. The Lord continues to protect all our friends in the four locations including Lacroix, where nothing usually happens anyway. The work continues with mission teams from France and elsewhere impacting communities throughout the nation of Haiti. For example, Pastor Michel Morriset has recently been named as the head of the Lions Club of Haiti. Their valuable work is helping with youth and other high-profile projects across the land.

The Lord has also expedited our applications for the new 501c3 mission organization and incorporation in the state of Oklahoma. It's official! We are now a nonprofit recognized by the Federal Government as "Vanguard Ministries International." Russ chose the title to symbolize our commitment to being on the front lines of the Gospel around the world.

We will once again partner with indigenous ministries to further God's kingdom. We want to continue our work with Eben-Ezer Mission in Haiti, a former partner in India working with tribals in the Eastern Ghat Mountains, and a new partnership with Peterson Outdoors Ministries in Missouri that works with disabled combat veterans and their families. Over the last six years Russ has had the privilege of gaining new friendships with many Hmong people now living in the US. After the end of the Vietnam War some of them emigrated from places such as Laos and Cambodia searching for freedom and a new life for their families.

Even if we can no longer live long-term in primitive conditions overseas, we can still do short-term training of pastors and lay people, hold conferences; sponsor vocational training, seek agricultural and engineering personnel to upgrade struggling ministries, and help send others to areas in need.

Afterword

An Invitation to Our Readers

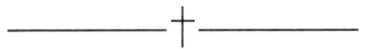

Every human being is separated from God because of sin. The Bible tells us, "But your iniquities have separated you from your God; and your sins have hidden His face from you, so that He will not hear." (Isaiah 59:2)

Many people may argue that, "I'm a good person. I haven't killed anyone. I've given to the poor, and go to church every Christmas and Easter. Surely, God wouldn't keep me out of heaven?" But the Bible also tells us, "For all of us have become like one who is unclean, and all our righteous deeds are like a filthy garment; And all of us wither like a leaf, And our iniquities, like the wind, take us away." (Isaiah 64:6)

Every living person has sinned. Romans 3:23 tells us, "… for all have sinned and fall short of the glory of God…" There is no one who has not sinned except Jesus Christ. The scriptures tell us, "There is no one righteous, not even one; there is no one who understands, no one who seeks God." (Romans 3:10-11)

And since we are separated from God because of our sin, there is only one way in this life to come to God. Jesus stated that, "I am the way and the truth and the life. No one comes to the Father except through me." (John 14:6)

Sin also separates us from:

1) Fellowship with God
2) The blessings of God, and
3) Some of the benefits of God's love.

Though God intended for us to have a relationship with Him, we naturally want to do things our own way. We're stubborn, selfish, and seldom able to follow through on our promises. Try as we might, we just keep stumbling. So, ultimately, because of our sin, we cannot know and experience God's love and plan for our life.

So how can we have a personal relationship with God?

Now, before sin can be forgiven, there must be a payment. That's right, there is a cost. Scripture tells us that, "…the wages of sin is death…" (Romans 6:23a). That is a pretty steep price. And it must be paid because that is what justice is all about. When we break the rules of this world, we must go before a judge in a court of law. If we are tried and found guilty we must be punished. The sin in our life means we have violated God's law, and therefore we must pay the penalty; a very steep penalty.

The penalty is DEATH!

Thankfully, God had a plan. And it could be accomplished only through His Son Jesus Christ. In His infinite wisdom, God knew this was not something we could do on our own. The Bible tells us this plan required someone to be crucified on a cross and to take our sins upon themselves. The only One perfect who could act as that sacrifice was Jesus Christ; the only One who could satisfy the demand of sin for justice.

So, one day "…God demonstrated His love toward us, in that, while we were still sinners, Christ died for us." (Romans 5:8) Christ went through much suffering for our sins. It is beyond our imagination what He endured. The human side of Christ knows exactly how we feel. He had the same feelings, the same sorrows, the same fears, and He experienced pain just like we do. He fully knows what it is to live a human life. On the Day of Judgment, no one will be able to point a finger at Christ and say, "You just don't know what it is to live as a human." Yes, He does. The dread, the fear, the sorrow, the mocking, the spitting, the pain of being beaten, and the crucifixion were all dreaded by our Lord. It hurt Him as much as it would us.

He was the innocent dying for us, the guilty.

Crucifixion on a cross was the cruelest form of torture that has ever been devised by man. There is nothing worse. Yet, our Lord allowed Himself to be taken up on that hill called Golgotha, nailed to a cross, and hung there in pain and agony for six long hours in a slow death, enduring punishment, so that God would save us.

What wonderful love, beyond description, that God and Christ have for us.

But that was not the end of it. After dying on that cruel cross, Jesus was buried in a stone cave. And after three days, He was gloriously raised from the dead and witnessed by the disciples and over five hundred people in various places and at various times. He Is Alive!

"Don't be alarmed," he said. "You are looking for Jesus the Nazarene, who was crucified. He has risen! He is not here. See the place where they laid him." (Mark 16:6)

The resurrection is a triumphant and glorious victory for every believer. Jesus Christ died, was buried, and rose the third day according to the Scripture. And, He is coming again! The dead in Christ will be raised up, and those who remain and are alive at His coming will be changed and receive new, glorified bodies.

"Brothers, we do not want you to be ignorant about those who fall asleep, or to grieve like the rest of men, who have no hope. We believe that Jesus died and rose again and so we believe that God will bring with Jesus those who have fallen asleep in him. According to the Lord's own word, we tell you that we who are still alive, who are left till the coming of the Lord, will certainly not precede those who have fallen asleep. For the Lord himself will come down from heaven, with a loud command, with the voice of the archangel and with the trumpet call of God, and the dead in Christ will rise first. After that, we who are still alive and are left will be caught up together with them in the clouds to meet the Lord in the air. And so we will be with the Lord forever." (1 Thessalonians 4:13-17)

Why is the resurrection of Jesus Christ important to salvation? The term "salvation" means being saved from death, which is the just punishment for our sins. The resurrection of Jesus from death demonstrated that God accepted Jesus' sacrifice on our behalf. It proves that God has the power to raise us from the dead. It guarantees that those who believe in Christ will not remain dead, but will be resurrected unto eternal life. That is our blessed hope!

So, how can we have this personal relationship with Jesus Christ and be forgiven of our sins?

To be forgiven, we must first accept that we are sinners and need to repent. Forgiveness is not automatic, but depends upon our confession of sin. "If we confess our sins, he is faithful and just and will forgive us our sins and purify us from all unrighteousness." (1 John 1:9)

There is no good work we can do to earn us a place in heaven, and we can take no credit for our salvation. "For it is by grace you have been saved, through faith—and this not from yourselves, it is the gift of God—not by works, so that no one can boast." (Ephesians 2:8-9)

When we confess Jesus as the living Lord we will never say anything more meaningful or as eternally important. Jesus was God in the flesh. No other religious leader, Moses, Buddha, and Muhammad, is His equal. They were simply men; Jesus is God who became a man. He is the center of all of life and creation. All of the world's greatest gifts, love, life, truth, and grace have a name. And that name is JESUS!

Now is the time to make things right with God. We invite you to confess your sinfulness by saying a simple prayer to God, and accept the sacrifice of Jesus Christ in your place. You were made for a person and a place. Jesus is the person, and heaven is the place. They are a package, they come together.

Allow me to leave you with one last thought. Isaiah 55:6 says, "Seek the LORD while he may be found; call on him while he is near." When you made this decision God has promised us, "Yet to all who received him, to those who believed in his name, he gave the right to become children of God." (John 1:12)

Call upon the Lord, and join me in praise and rejoicing to the God of Heaven for all eternity!

I look forward to seeing you there.

We invite you to partner with us to advance the Gospel of our Lord Jesus Christ, alleviate poverty and hopelessness, and help spread the joy of the Lord across the world!

Be part of the Vanguard:

Vanguard Ministries International
PO Box 1895, Stillwater OK 74076
vmi2019@protonmail.com

Printed in the USA
CPSIA information can be obtained
at www.ICGtesting.com
LVHW060201090124
768419LV00055B/1151